LETHAL DOSE

ONE MAN'S JOURNEY THROUGH A PHASE 1 DRUG TRIAL

LETHAL DOSE

ONE MAN'S JOURNEY THROUGH A PHASE 1 DRUG TRIAL

PAT MADDOCKS

Introduction

Dear Reader,

This book was written out of devotion and desperation. I never wanted to involve the media nor burden you with the story of my husband, Dave's, harrowing experience as a test subject in a drug trial. You have been disillusioned enough by exposés of the lack of integrity in high places.

Shortly after Dave's death, once I'd scraped myself off the floor, and with help from family and friends, I started a campaign to improve the monitoring and medical care of Phase I participants. We began by directing our well-documented concerns to the executives of the many bureaucracies involved. The powers-that-be threw us some legally vetted reports containing measured apologetic phrases and reassurances that the protocols already in place were entirely adequate. Their reports further assured us that these rules of conduct would, *now*, be strictly followed. They then circled their wagons and severed communications. We've persisted on alternate fronts, but the reality is, the medical research establishment isn't motivated to change its ways; the status quo works nicely — for them. You are our final court of appeal.

There is a simple reason why the medical research industry can dismiss the issues that Dave's case has spotlighted: their governing body — our society — is oblivious to the actual workings of the drug development process. Secrecy has long been a tool used by elitist groups to protect their influence and power. Like so many of us, Dave and I coasted along, assuming that the medical profession still adhered to its age-old solemn oath to "Do No Harm." Sadly, as Oscar Wilde has said, "When you 'assume,' you make an 'ass' out of 'u' and 'me.'"

Lethal Dose will educate you about what happens in the evolution of a new drug after the testing on lab animals is completed. This book is an intimate account of Dave's recruitment and experiences throughout a Phase I cancer clinical trial. The focus of this narrative is not the drug, but Dave, the person.

Please read on ...

Regards,

Patricia Maddocks
June 16, 2011

Bear Ring "U" 'n Mind Foundation
*Research *with* Respect*

Throughout Lethal Dose, *pseudonyms have been substituted for the names of those medical people intrinsic to Dave's story. My lawyers have deemed this necessary to mitigate possible libel action. For the same reason, descriptive adjectives have been kept to a minimum. At this point, I consider it a mixed blessing that I have a good memory for conversations. Nonetheless, that personal attribute has been invaluable, especially during my hundreds of hours volunteering on a local crisis line and while assembling this book. If the phrasing of an exchange between characters jars, rest easy: the content is correct.*

Library and Archives Canada Cataloguing in Publication

Maddocks, Pat, 1944 –
Lethal dose : one man's journey through a phase 1 drug trial / Pat Maddocks.

Includes bibliographical references.
Also issued in electronic format.
ISBN 978-0-9868952-0-3

1. Maddocks, Dave, 1936 – 2005. 2. Drugs — Testing.
3. Cancer — Patients — Canada — Biography. I. Title.

RM301.27.M33 2011 616.9940610724 C2011-905178-8

Cover photograph by Dave Maddocks

Contents

THIS BOOK IS DEDICATED TO ALL THOSE WHO PROVIDE CARE AND TO ALL THOSE WHO NEED IT.

"Hope is disappointment postponed."

Dr. Laura Schlessinger and
Rabbi Stewart Vogel

CHAPTER ONE
Sweating
JANUARY 2006

It's a moment she would never have imagined for herself: standing half-naked and distraught in front of their bedroom window, alone in their house, getting dressed for a sweat lodge ceremony to honour her husband. Pat looks out over Springhill Farm as she pulls on her outfit — a sea-blue *salwar kameez*, the cotton breezy and soft, the neckline of the tunic framed by tiny mirrors and sequins. This magnificent view that they carved out of scrub alders, this massive house that they created together — they are the only things keeping her grounded these days. Despite the comfort of the familiar blanket of green fields spread out below her, she feels light-headed, shaky, overcome with sadness.

Wrapping the billowing scarf around her shoulders, she thinks of how perfectly these clothes cover her birthmark — the port-wine stain snaking all the way from her chest down one arm to her fingertips, her wedding rings sparkling against purple skin. She smiles, remembering when she bought this traditional Indian outfit several years earlier on a cruise from Auckland to Venice. Back then, she couldn't have anticipated having an opportunity to wear it. She bought it on a whim, caught up in the frenzy of a charity auction, certain it was a good cause but an entirely impractical purchase.

Of course, Dave knew it was the voluminous scarf she liked, not the rest of the outfit. In the crowded ballroom, she had kept pushing up the bidding. And he'd laughed and given her a huge bear hug when she'd sheepishly signaled with her eyes and a shrug of her shoulders that she'd been the winner. Later, at the bar, with a knowing sparkle in his big, brown eyes, he'd clinked her glass. "To silliness, Bridget!" he said. "Thanks, Sid!" she'd responded wryly. Instead of "dear" or "darling," they'd slipped onto this comfortable habit of using their middle names for endearment, especially in public; their discreet form of shared intimacy and support.

Standing here now in that impractical outfit, she thinks about how she would never have considered a sweat lodge ceremony before Dave died and everything changed. Now, here in their bedroom, she feels like a stranger in her own life.

She has to squint to stop the tears, to steel herself for the night ahead. She will soon be joining a group of people she doesn't know, in a ceremony she doesn't understand. But what she wants most is to reverse the tide of time, to stop replaying the horror of Dave's last week in her mind, to stop the constant feeling of dread. She so wants her husband back.

The setting sun is turning the sky a pastel pink, and the not-so-distant snow-capped mountains are a soft blue. The fields of the farm she bought with Dave 28 years earlier undulate gently down towards the highway. In the middle of this familiar vista is their treasured giant maple, its bare branches etched in stark relief against the darkening winter sky.

Cold night air sweeps over Pat as she walks out their front door and across the gravel driveway towards the sweat lodge that their basement suite tenant, Phil, has built in the middle of their 14 acres of West Coast woodland. Phil's four wolves, all members of the same pack, pace the perimeter of the high wire fence that encloses their acre of forest. She steps off the manicured lawn, pushing through the squeaky wooden gate onto the trail, the earth spongy underfoot. Breathing in the scent of wet earth and Douglas fir, she suddenly wants to turn around, to go back home and collapse on their bed. But she has agreed to come to this ceremony, to participate in a tribute of respect to her dead husband.

At the end of the trail, Phil is waiting, his long, brown hair pulled into a ponytail, his face warm and welcoming. Their long-term tenant and friend, he stands in front of a huge, crackling fire in which small boulders are heating up. His eyes meet hers and immediately Pat is at ease. She feels at once silly and solemn. There is nothing further from her conservative, traditional Catholic upbringing than this tarp-covered domed structure in the woods. But she welcomes the chance to be pushed out of her comfort zone.

Standing in the darkening woods, the fire blazing, she is flooded with guilt and with disappointment in herself. It has been almost a month since Dave died, and she has tried every day, in vain, to find a way to talk to him, to apologize. She is questioning the Christian notion that Dave is now up in the sky with God on his throne surrounded by angels. She has immersed herself in the *Tibetan Book of the Dead* and is struggling to define her own version of the afterlife. She knows energy doesn't just disappear; it becomes something else. She knows Dave's life force is out there. That he might be part of someone or something else.

Rubbing her hands in front of the fire, Pat looks around at what Phil has built in this clearing on their property. Neither Dave nor Pat knew this sweat lodge existed. They thought Phil had built some type of shelter for his wolves. Nothing like this. It's a round, womb-like structure constructed from cedar boughs and covered with layers of blankets and a tarp. Dave, she thinks to herself, would be smiling if he could see his wife here now. Behind the fire is a primitive altar — a large, twisting wooden stick enshrined with animal skulls and shells. On a mossy stump, at the base of the stick, are candles, fresh flowers, bunches of sage and sweet grass, and a ceremonial pipe.

Phil quietly explains that the stones being heated in the fire are volcanic "grandfather" rocks that come from all over North

America and that he'll be bringing them into the sweat lodge seven at a time, four times, over the course of the two-hour session. There are 28 ribs in the buffalo, the animal revered by the Lakota people, which is why the numbers 4 and 7 and their multiples are considered to be sacred. This, says Phil, is a White Buffalo Peace Pipe Ceremony.

Pat can't help smiling, thinking how Dave would laugh at the idea of bringing rocks onto the property. He had spent a lot of time clearing land. One of Dave's favourite toys was a huge, hydraulic rock picker that could sift the soil and carry a ton of rocks at a time. Dave had gone over all 65 arable acres of Springhill several times and had even done custom work removing rocks for the Parks Board and other farmers. Hauling rocks in? Totally ironic!

Pat returns her gaze to Phil. He lights a bunch of sweet grass and wafts the smoke over her body, hair and face. She is ready.

She crouches to enter the lodge through a small flap. On the floor inside are more blankets — bright yellows, reds and blues — and beneath them are freshly picked swordferns that provide a softening shield from the hard earth. In the darkness, she looks up and sees Phil's medicine wheel: a round, leather-bound dream catcher the size of a record album, hanging from the centre of the lodge, with feathers dangling from its web-like strings.

More people come in through the flap but she doesn't pay attention. She doesn't want to connect with people these days. And now, in here, she feels more blessedly alone than ever. She wants desperately to make this a penance, an act of contrition. She knows little of the ceremony except that it will get unbearably and painfully hot. She desires this pain; maybe her suffering will make partial amends to Dave.

Seven "grandfathers" are passed by pitchfork into the earthen pit at the centre of the lodge. Then the flap closes. Now the darkness is absolute, causing Pat to catch her breath. She vaguely senses the 10 or so people beside her, but she can't see them. She can't see anything. She is blind. She closes her eyes. Breathes in the scent of musky earth and rising heat. Listens to Phil's drumming and his voice softly chanting.

When Pat opens her eyes again, she can see a bit more of the interior. She inhales the sweet, smoky mist rising from the sage and sweet grass that spontaneously combusts as it is placed on the heated stones. Phil sprinkles fine cedar shavings into the pit and sparks fly into the blackness like miniature fireworks. She hears the crackling of water being poured over the rocks, and she notices the rocks are glowing — a deep, blood red.

Suddenly, like an assault, there is the image of blood pouring out of Dave's nose and mouth. She closes her eyes again, clenches her teeth. She sees herself grappling with the little metal bowl in the emergency ward. His blood spilling into the small, shiny dish, splattering onto her jeans. She can't stop the vision. She is back with him in the hospital, holding his dying body, stroking his hands.

The blood is so shocking; it had started while she was looking the other way, talking to their daughter Michele. She thinks to herself, "I took my eyes off of him! There I was talking to somebody else, not paying attention, and he was taking his last breath." She berates herself for her inattention. *Mea culpa*, she pleads, reverting to her Catholic roots. *Mea maxima culpa*.

Without knowing it, she has prayed this out loud. She is asked to speak, to put her greatest need into words: "I'm so sorry, Dave. I truly didn't realize you were dying. Forgive me for begging you to try harder, to stay with me. It was so wrong. I knew you were trying as hard as you could."

She feels the sweat dripping down her back. It is hard to breathe. She wants to leave, crawl for the flap, but she stays rooted to the floor. Instead, she grabs her towel and wipes the sweat that is dripping down her face. Others in the tent are talking now, taking turns sharing their stories. The talking circle is an integral part of the sweat ceremony and everyone is invited to share their grief, their pain. Someone is speaking about their child's problem with drugs. Phil talks too, about his anxiety over his son leaving soon for Afghanistan to serve in the army.

"But it doesn't matter how bad things are," says Phil. "There is always something to be grateful for."

Pat feels the sweat mixing with tears running down her cheeks. She is thinking about how grateful she is for the life she had with Dave. For all the happy memories he has left her. She sees his face now in the moments after his death. She remembers how beautiful he was. How handsome, with that deep cleft in his chin, his strong, angular jaw, his bushy eyebrows and his big, brown eyes.

Phil's voice goes wobbly, and Pat starts to feel dizzy. She fumbles for a water bottle and drinks deeply. She lies down on her side, her head against the ground. She pulls back the blanket and fern carpeting and turns her face to the earth, her cheek and hands touching the bare soil, trying to absorb its cool wetness. The drums beat on. Voices rise in song.

The flap opens and seven more rocks are passed in with a pitchfork. Pat realizes she is only one quarter of the way through the ceremony and her senses rebel. Her mind is flooded with the recollection of returning home to Courtenay a few days after his death.She remembers rinsing her bloody jeans in the big metal bowl she usually reserved for making potato salad. The blood turned the water pale pink and she walked out into their backyard and poured it all onto the base of the giant maple that framed their view of the farm.

Dave loved that tree. He spent so many hours photographing its stark winter beauty, its ever-changing seasonal outfits. They never took the time to relax in the shade of that tree, Pat thinks sadly. They were too busy running the farm, and later, managing their other properties between serious travel expeditions.

She tunes back in to Phil's voice. He is talking about Dave. "So much of Dave was about the land," he says. "This land we're sitting on was such a huge part of him. All his energy, focus and work. His tractors, irrigation systems, rakes and hoes. This land is steeped with his spirit. He was physically connected to this place and this place with him."

The flap opens again and the cold air rushes in. Pat breathes in the relief and watches them pass in seven more rocks. She tries to focus on gratitude, on happy memories. He always took such exquisite care of her. But then she is crushed with guilt, for she believes she does not deserve happiness. In the heat of the darkness, Dave keeps coming back to her in bits of moving images: light through the trees, boots clomping through the mud on their farm, his hands on the tractor.

Then, scenes from Dave's final hours flash before her: his blackened feet, his limp, quivering body, his panic when she tried to shade his eyes from the glare of the fluorescent hospital lights with a face cloth, his ragged breathing, the kidney specialist who said there was nothing more they could do.

Nothing more. Her sweat feels like heavy drops of water, like tears. "We didn't get the chance to say goodbye, Sid," she thinks to herself. "I lost you. I tried to hold on, but I lost you."

Pat feels her body sinking into the cold earth. Since Dave's death her grief has been a heavy stone in her chest. Now the heaviness becomes resolve. She makes one more wifely vow: "I will find out the truth so that we both may rest in peace."

CHAPTER TWO

Farming

AUGUST 1984

It's 5:00 a.m. and Pat blinks awake. The early morning light is her alarm clock. She slips softly from their double bed, careful not to wake Dave; he'd been welding the potato combine until after midnight. She grabs her clothes and tiptoes down the hallway to the bathroom. Once dressed, she nukes a mug of half milk, half leftover coffee, careful to stop the microwave before the buzzer goes off. She sips quickly and gratefully before heading out onto the farm.

It's August, the height of summer, but just lately the early mornings are quite cool. She tucks her grey work socks into yellow gumboots, puts on her red and grey plaid work jacket — the one that used to be Dave's — and grabs her black rubber gloves. The gravel crunches under her feet as she sets off to get her favourite of their six tractors, the Massey Ferguson with its running board low to the ground. The farm is just waking up: the 800 laying hens are clucking as they peck through their earthen enclosure, the pygmy goats are bleating softly. She can hear in the distance the low rumbling of the occasional vehicle passing by on the highway.

In the machinery shed, Pat is all business. She revs up the Massey and takes it over to the fuel tank to gas it up before heading out to the fields. She passes the acre-long hills of red Pontiac potatoes, a sea of green topped with rose-pink flowers fanning up the gentle slope. She passes row upon row of peaches and cream corn in full tassel; the tangled forest of asparagus, their stalks now tall, lacy fronds twinkling with dew; the harvested hectare of English peas with yellowed vines that Dave had trimmed to the ground with the brush-cutter. She shakes her head. Just a week ago, that pea field had been further flattened by the hundreds of cars parked on it. Springhill had a huge turnout, 7,000 visitors — a new record — for the annual "Tour the Farms" event. What a zoo! Thank heaven for their energetic family, friends and staff who had done such a fabulous job of pitching in to organize, entertain and feed that fun-seeking mob of day trippers.

She pulls into the broccoli field, hops off the tractor, rummages in the tool box on the tractor's fender for her special thin-bladed knife that Dave has yet again sharpened for her, and grabs her first bucket. She walks up and down the long rows, slicing off the dark green domes.

Thoughts of their daughters pop into her head, both so far away, Lisa on a Rotary scholarship in Japan, Michele volunteering with Canada World Youth in Somalia. She and Dave had planned to make a quick dash to both countries late this fall to see the girls and bring them Christmas goodies. But they won't be able to visit Michele; the Canadian embassy has issued a travel advisory saying that, due to rampant civil unrest, it couldn't sanction tourists traveling to Somalia. That only served to increase their concerns for their eldest daughter. Pat will talk to Dave about organizing the trip to Yamaguchi, to visit Lisa. He is the travel junkie and will be keen to get something booked. So much needs to be done, though, just to get away for three weeks. Springhill's 65 acres of veggies, plus its acre and a half of greenhouse crops, are so demanding. December is the least hectic month in the farm year. They can be away during those weeks only because Mary Curnew, their marvelous retail sales manager, and her husband are willing to take over running the veggie stand, to stock and man it all seven days of the week. By January 1, Dave and Pat must be back to start planting the greenhouse crops.

Despite the seemingly endless mental list of things to do, Pat smiles. It strikes her that she is living exactly the life she always wanted: working, playing, dreaming, scheming, every day, alongside her husband. With the 16 five-gallon buckets full of broccoli crowns, she heads back to the house for a bite of breakfast.

Springhill has been good to them. Back in 1978 when they'd come to Courtenay, a small city on the east coast of Vancouver Island, they weren't sure it was the right place to start another farming venture. Courtenay was on the cusp of being too far north, increasing the risk of a too-short growing season. They had thought Nanaimo would be best, being at the centre of the Island and with a larger customer base, but there was no farmland suitable for veggie crops on the market then.

So she and Dave traveled up to Courtenay where they had pre-arranged with an agent to show them what was for sale in the Comox Valley. Driving up the old Island highway, they'd passed breathtaking ocean views and rambling farmland. The real estate agent knew what they wanted: something small and manageable, maybe 20 arable acres, ideally with an opportunity to rent more land in the immediate area.

The agent showed them several properties, all with obvious drawbacks — first, one with swamp grass–infested fields, then another with very limited water supply. But late in the afternoon, he drove them to Springhill Farm, identified by a poky white sign swinging on a stick of steel. The snow-capped mountains of the Beaufort Range seemed just an arm's length away. The rugged peak of the Mount Washington ski "hill" glistened in the sun as the realtor's car inched along the quarter-mile gravel lane that led to a dingy, dirt-brown, shingled house.

The disused dairy barn, the machinery sheds, the workshop: they all screamed neglect and decay. Dave and Pat almost gave Springhill the thumbs down. At 112 acres, with only 40 acres of that cleared, it was about five times too big. But though

Springhill was battered, it was still beautiful: gently sloping southwest exposure, 10 minutes from town, and a fabulous water supply of two reservoirs, one so big the locals called it Shannon Lake.

The realtor persuaded Dave to walk the fields. So Dave grabbed his soil probe and headed out. He randomly plunged the probe into the sandy loam, no less than 30 times, and didn't hit a single rock or stone (although he did later!). That's when they knew they were hooked. Mr. Clark, the elderly owner, was happy to give his permission for the use of the Springhill Farm name and keen to see it revitalized by Dave's plans for the property. Their offer was accepted and the deal was sealed.

Within a few years, they were growing everything from A to Z — asparagus to zucchini, asters to zinnias. By the highway, they hung out a big yellow sign with a large painting of a potato plant. Alongside, Dave set up a steel frame with slots to slide in the names of the crops currently available. But that was only a teaser. There were so many crops, especially in the summer, that they couldn't possibly advertise them all. They grew 36 varieties of vegetables, either seeded directly into the ground or produced from the millions of transplants they'd propagated and set out every two weeks during the growing season. One new crop a year: that was their motto. Nowadays, they have about 30 employees and a market garden that draws hundreds of eager customers daily.

Dave is up, making coffee. "Good morning," they say in unison as they give each other a quick hug and their signature kiss — two tender teasing pecks and a long lip lock. Smiling as she draws him over to the kitchen window, she says, "Sid, look at the twins you delivered last week." Across the lawn, next to the refurbished red dairy barn, is one of Dave's impulse buys — a group of black and white pygmy goats. They're chasing each other around their pen, racing up and down the series of ramps he's built for them. The little tribe is a huge hit and a surprising boost to Springhill's coffers. The customers and especially their children eagerly feed the cute animals after putting quarters in the grain-filled gumball machine that Dave has installed on a fence post. Dave chuckles as the babies suddenly zip up to their mother and bunt her udder, searching for their breakfast.

But the quiet moment is interrupted by the slamming of car doors, announcing the 7:30 a.m. arrival of Springhill's staff.

The workers filter into the farmhouse kitchen for the usual morning meeting and assignment of tasks, helping themselves to coffee. Pat looks over at her husband, totally engrossed in bantering "tech talk" with his crew. He's so capable, a practical genius. She takes in his chiseled jawline and sexy cleft chin, his gentle, brown eyes, his wide smile, his deep, gravelly voice. Twenty-one years of marriage and she's still madly in love.

They met when she was a junior high school student in their hometown of Richmond, an urban agricultural community outside of Vancouver. For several summers, she'd picked strawberries and raspberries at Twin Hollies, the farm owned by Dave's family. He was 22 and she 14 when she first saw him, the youngest in a family of nine children. He was gorgeous with his buzz cut and honey-coloured skin. But Pat never thought he'd even noticed her, not surrounded by the hundreds of teenage girls in their skimpy summer clothes. She was always wearing long-sleeve shirts with a buttoned-up collar to cover her purple birthmark.

Dave was like James Dean with his Levi's and T-shirt and his pack of Export 'A' cigarettes rolled up in his sleeve. As farm manager, he'd bomb around his parent's 200-acre dairy, berry and potato operation in his little green Austin, a cigarette dangling from his mouth, the girls swooning over him.

Three summers after first meeting Dave, when Pat had just graduated from high school, she was waiting for her dad to pick her up on his way home from work. The Twin Hollies field supervisor had given Pat the message that her dad, the CEO of the local credit union, was going to be very late.

As Dave drove by in the old army truck that he used to transport the berry pickers, he braked suddenly and hollered down from the cab asking if she'd like to come along for the ride. She had to hide her surprise. "Sure," she remembers saying, trying to be casual.

She had never been in a troop truck before and suppressed her excitement as she sat beside him, the workers on the benches in the back. The hot summer air blew at her face as he drove to several day-labourer assembly points in south Vancouver to drop off his passengers. Occasionally, he would turn to her and smile. The roar of the motor didn't give much opportunity for conversation. The truck was too big to drive into her Richmond subdivision, so he let her off at the top of the road leading to her house. Her four younger brothers and sisters were playing on the lawn as she arrived home. They screamed at her to join them, but she was in another world, her bright blue-grey eyes ablaze with a new enchantment.

He officially proposed to her three months later at the base of Grouse Mountain. While he considerately held a flashlight so she could see the exquisite ring in the darkness of his car, the lights of the city twinkling beyond, she knew she would be in love with this man as long as she lived. She was so happy that he had agreed to choose her engagement ring: it was dainty, just as she had wanted, a perfectly lovely 18th birthday present. A couple of months earlier, when he had first talked about them getting married, Pat suggested that perhaps she was kind of young, that maybe they should wait for a while. But Dave was convinced otherwise. He had saved up money to travel around Europe and he told her he was going to hit the road if she didn't agree to marry him. He added that he had no idea when he would return, and he wasn't much of a letter writer. Pat knew she wanted to marry Dave and, despite her young age, she knew exactly what she wanted — a husband she could work with, and be with, every minute of every day.

At Springhill, that's exactly what has happened. They spend

hours together — clearing land; cultivating fields; planting and harvesting crops; washing, grading and packaging potatoes, carrots and a myriad of other field crops; pruning, harvesting and packaging greenhouse crops of tomatoes, peppers and kiwis and shrink-wrapping long English cucumbers. They set up sales displays, determine prices, debate which varieties of seeds to order and make treks to the Mainland to pick up supplies.

Dave's ingenuity and determination turned a marginal enterprise into a million-dollar-a-year business. He has put the word "profitable" back into farming. Dave also believes in supporting other local entrepreneurs. Springhill sells their frozen emu meat, fresh-baked bread from home-ground wheat, locally pressed apple juice, pies and other baked goodies, relishes, jams and honeys — helping bolster their businesses and enhancing Springhill's cornucopia of top-quality produce.

While Dave spends most of his time managing crops and maintaining machinery and buildings, Pat looks after their staff and public relations, often greeting customers and introducing them to new food ideas. Today, she's going to talk up the delicious taste of raw rutabaga, offering shoppers a plate of julienne strips. She'll also be promoting raw corn. Dave is fond of saying that Nature gives corn the perfect packaging and it riles him when customers willy-nilly tear it open. As soon as corn is exposed to the air, its sugars start turning to starch. So to ease Dave's angst, Pat attempts to minimize any "dinner-rush" ripping by taking a torn and rejected cob out of the bin and, with an Exacto knife, slicing off a block of the crisp kernels onto her surgical-gloved hand. She does all this right in front of the gaggle of people gathered around the display.

With an inviting grin, she asks the now curious customers, "Have you had your corn flakes today?" The shoppers hesitantly put out their hands for a sample. Pat is always amazed by how few people have ever tried raw corn. Invariably, exclamations of

"Hey, this is really good!" result and Pat then gives simple hints on how to choose an ear of corn — without ripping the wrappings. On days when she can fit in time to put on this bit of street theatre, the number of trashed cobs is greatly reduced.

This morning, as they have every day for the past month, the crew will be harvesting pickling cucumbers. Two acres of them. It's a back-breaking job. The dark green cucumbers hide under miles of creeping vines with their masses of huge, prickly leaves hugging the ground. If the pickers don't get them at exactly the right size, just one more day could make them too large for dill pickles. Then the "cukes" become the lower-valued bread-and-butter size.

Dave and Pat confer with Mary, Springhill's market manager. Together they decide what's needed from the fields and greenhouses to keep her display counters up. Dave announces that the ninth planting of cauliflower needs to be cut and that the yellow sticky bug traps in the carrot fields are due to be collected and replaced. He asks Pat to distribute this week's shipment of biologicals — "good bugs" just dropped off by Loomis — throughout the greenhouses. Wherever possible, Dave has implemented Integrated Pest Management (IPM) strategies. Steve, Mary's husband, is dispatched to spot the five-gallon buckets for the pickle pickers. Then he will harvest several totes of each kind of lettuce before he starts on the cauliflower, ending his day seeing to the sticky traps. After pickles, some of the crew will pick green and wax beans. Some will weed and hoe the pumpkin patch. Some will snap the tops off the super-tender Nantes carrots. But first Dave will loosen the crop with his ingenious, self-made carrot-bed lifter, which makes it so much easier for the crew to pull out the carrots. Pat and Dave orchestrate Springhill, a symphony they compose and conduct together.

"I've got to spray the turnips with boron before the wind comes up," says Dave as he heads out the door. "Let's go, people. Smile, it's showtime."

Everyone files out of the house to start working in the fields, in the greenhouses, in the market or in the potato pit to package produce. Dave will change tractors, collect the freshly picked pickling cukes and begin washing, grading and packaging them into 10-pound bags. It's not unusual to sell 2,000 pounds a day.

Customers start arriving by 9:00 a.m., driving up the long, gravel road into the middle of the farm and parking in front of the long, low, barn-red veggie stand. Now the height of summer, their market is all but obscured by millions of blossoms. Dave's innovative watering and fertilizing system ensures that the building's roof and support posts are outlined — spring, summer and fall — with vibrant flowers and healthy plants. At this time of year, the overflowing tiers of red cascading ivy geraniums are a show-stopper. Customers are always looking up in awe.

By mid-afternoon, it's time to pick yet another bin of corn, a task that is done four or five times a day. Customers love to see the tractors roaring in from the fields, totes loaded with just-picked buckets of corn. Today that's Pat's job and she hops back onto the Massey, drives past the potato fields and right into the tall stalks of corn that have already been harvested. She sees that a large swath of corn stalks has been decimated, a mess of shredded cobs on the dirt. She swears under her breath, "Blasted raccoons!"

She walks among the towering plants, her left hand grabbing each stalk below the ear of corn — there's usually only one cob per plant — then her right hand yanking down on the ear to snap it off. Buckets full and stacked into the plywood tote, she steps back onto her tractor and throws her leg over the seat. Just as she's getting comfortable, she sees it — a big, black lump straight ahead.

It's a bear, lying fast asleep in the cornfield. Startled, muttering "shit, shit shit!" under her breath, she slams the gearshift into reverse and backs down the rough track before the bear moves. Dave is rototilling in the next field. She waves him down.

"Dave," she shouts. "I almost ran over a bear sleeping in the cornfield!"

"Damn," he responds. "Are you okay?"

They both know bears like corn just as much as people and raccoons do. Pat is calmer now and jokes that the bear was just like Dave. "You like to have a snooze after pigging out on corn too," she laughs.

Dave says that with the commotion of her gunning the tractor, the bear will be gone by now. "They don't mix with people, if they can help it. Have you got enough corn to cover the five o'clock rush?"

"No," she replies. "I'll have to go back later."

Dave offers to do the last run, but Pat assures him she can do it.

"Well, make lots of noise going in and keep making noise while you're picking," he advises.

When she goes back, she bangs her buckets loudly and sings, over and over again, at the top of her lungs. "N-E-S-T-L-E-S. Nestles makes the very best ... chocolate." The ad jingle is all she can think of. She hopes the bear is gone. It is. The next day, Dave attaches a bicycle horn onto the Massey. "Let 'em know you're coming, Bridget," he laughs.

It's just after six; the last customers and market staff have gone home. Dave and Pat pack up the veggie stand, cash out the tills and walk across the lawn to the house for a quick dinner of corn on the cob. But their day doesn't end until well after sundown. The TV news and dinner digested, Dave heads back to the fields to move the irrigation systems, repositioning the traveling sprinkler guns and setting up the hand lines. Pat goes to work cutting flowers for the mixed bouquets that are sold in the market. With the flowers nestled in their buckets of water and tucked away in the refrigerated potato pit for the night, Pat settles into a chair on the patio to wait for Dave.

The sky is turning turquoise and pink, and she can hear the birds chittering in the tall fir trees that surround the old farmhouse. It's country quiet again. At last.

When she looks up, she sees him. Striding down the gently sloping hillside in his big black rubber boots, his green workshirt hanging out of his jeans, the shirttails flapping in the warm evening breeze. The cottonwood trees behind him are lit up, their lime green leaves burnished to gold in the setting sun. He stops at the top of a potato field to turn on the water. The mist from the irrigation line sends off sparkles of rainbows and she watches them land on Dave's shoulders as he walks on through the arc of water towards the farmhouse.

Watching him approach, she is still breathless, even after all these years. He must be bushed, yet his every step is solid, deliberate, confident. He looks up and their eyes meet across the distance. Pat smiles, her pulse quickening.

CHAPTER 3
Stumbling
AUGUST 2005

It's a different Dave that Pat sees outside her kitchen window now. A different view, too. They are living in the ranch house just above the farm, overlooking the wide expanse of fields. They built this house on the hill so they could retire from farming but continue to live overlooking the land they love.

Outside the kitchen window, Pat can see the giant maple, its green branches stretching out into the clear summer sky. A mere skiff of snow remains on the highest mountain peaks in the distance. She is looking for Dave, who went out earlier for a walk, but she can't see him. Just a month ago, they returned from a two-month cruise around Europe from Rome to Berlin. This morning, Dave had suggested hiking the back trails of the farm, to check out the water levels in the reservoirs. Pat was surprised that he had the energy. He is more tired than usual these days. But most of Springhill is no longer their farm to walk upon freely. They sold over 90 acres of it two years ago.

"Those parts of the farm aren't ours anymore, Sid," Pat had told him. "I don't want to go. You go if you're so curious. I'll stay here and make lunch."

Pat is now busy making his favourite meal: sausage pie and creamed corn. But it's already past 1:00 p.m., their regular lunch time and Dave has been gone more than two hours. She is getting worried. She goes out to the glassed-in deck overlooking the farm, drying her hands on a tea towel, squinting into the sun to find Dave. She can see the ducks on the reservoir, their waterfront. Her favourite wild duck, a goldeneye with white and black feathers, is preening himself in the water. She looks out at the fields rolling down to the highway, the little, white farmhouse, the old barn, the glistening domes of empty greenhouses.

And then she spots him, in amongst the tangle of Scotch broom that engulfs the fence and the gate at the bottom of the grassy hill separating their house from the farm's back forty. Pushing open the gate, he sprawls forward. A small smile crosses her face. He must have tripped on the strand of barbed wire that runs along the bottom, she thinks. She sees him try to get up, but he falls down. He tries again, takes a small step and again falls. Then, shockingly, he begins to crawl on all fours up the gentle slope. She can now see that he is soaked. Stunned, Pat is momentarily paralyzed. Finally, gathering her wits, she runs through the house and out the side door to get to him. But when she opens the door, he is already there. She helps him into the house and sits him down in his leather recliner. His face is ashen, he is drenched in sweat, his breathing ragged and uneven.

"What the heck happened to you?" Pat asks.

"I collapsed in the trees by the lower reservoir," he gasps. "And I was too weak to get back up. I had to crawl most of the way up the lane. I barely made it."

"Did you have your Ventolin puffer with you?" asks Pat. "Did you use it?"

Dave nods his head.

"That didn't help?" she says, surprised.

"Mmm," he mumbles.

He struggles to breathe, wheezing, so she stifles the urge to ask more questions. A while later, she suggests going to the walk-in clinic.

"You need to see a doctor," she says. But Dave assures her

that he feels okay now, promising that he will tell Dr. Wilbur all about this episode when he sees him for his annual physical in a few days.

* * * * *

Dave's health has been compromised for years. But even with the seizures and his difficulty with breathing, he has managed to live a normal retired life — maintaining their house and yard, visiting his girls and their five grandchildren, traveling and cruising.

Fifteen years earlier, he'd had several silent heart attacks that had destroyed his left ventricle. Quintuple bypass surgery had helped, but the domino-effect damage to his lungs was irreparable. He was diagnosed with Chronic Obstructive Pulmonary Disease, or COPD. The medications for COPD, particularly prednisone, work to keep him breathing but also come with long-term, harmful side effects to his organs. Then he developed pulmonary embolisms and then esophageal ulcers, and his list of medications kept growing. Dave dealt with it all diligently, meticulous about arranging the pills by time and date in their own proper little plastic vials. To Pat, his medicine cabinet was a work of art. Despite all this, their lives had rolled along smoothly. Until now.

On their recent cruise, Dave had had another seizure. Pat called them "meltdowns" and, despite several investigations, no one knew what they were or why they happened. At least five times a year, for more than 17 years, Dave would be roused from a deep sleep with a really high fever and the shakes. He would feel so cold. The only thing that helped was a long soak in a warm bath. These attacks could go on for hours, leaving him weak and exhausted, his muscles like jelly. The next day, he would be back to normal.

The first time it happened, they were in a hotel room in Hong Kong. They attributed it to bad seafood. Back home, standard blood tests found nothing. At one point, their doctor thought it was malaria. When that didn't pan out, the doctor suggested getting to the emergency department while an attack was in progress. But when they got there, the ER was too busy to draw blood and Dave was shunted to a gurney in the hallway. When he was finally attended to, 10 hours later, the symptoms had ceased. After that frustrating episode, Pat could not persuade Dave to pursue any further testing.

When a seizure came on midway through their last European cruise, Pat knew how to handle things. They were docked in Copenhagen, and Dave was disappointed he was going to miss that port of call. He had arranged to meet a friend of a friend; instead, he spent most of the day in their stateroom bathtub trying to warm his body and recover. As usual, he was fine the next day and managed to get off the ship at Stockholm for a tour. It wasn't until much later that Pat realized those seizures might have been the first clues.

* * * * *

A few days after Pat finds Dave crawling up the hill, it is their 42nd wedding anniversary. Before going to the doctor for Dave's checkup, they decide to stop at the local Japanese restaurant for lunch — their anniversary ritual. Over sushi and tea, Pat can't help thinking about all the seizures. They have to mean something. But what? How could all those blood tests come up with nothing?

At the medical clinic later that day Dave and Pat are ushered into Dr. Wilbur's office. He has been Dave's doctor for a couple of decades and is showing signs of burnout, but masks it with hearty informality. Dr. Wilbur usually likes to start patient visits with a glib preamble, but foregoes the routine this time and immediately comments on Dave's pallor. His observation floors Pat, and reminds her that her sister and daughter had both recently commented that Dave was looking unusually pale. After his physical and a review of his medications, Dr. Wilbur gives Dave a requisition for some blood tests.

When Dr. Wilbur telephones on the weekend with the results, he says Dave's hemoglobin of 80 is way too low and he will need two sessions of blood transfusions. He says he's concerned Dave might be losing blood internally but that the transfusions should help with his fatigue. It is a sombre Sunday drive to St. Joseph's Hospital, past the Air Park, the church and Comox Inlet with its herons and beached rowboats.

They enter the squat building through the sliding glass doors, the summer breeze mixing with the hospital's stale air conditioning. At the end of the hallway, they are escorted to the transfusion room, and there they sit in hard, leather chairs, looking out over the ocean and the mountains, waiting for new blood, an injection of energy, a cure for the exhaustion Dave is feeling. The nurse tells Dave that Dr. Wilbur wants stool samples and Pat goes down to the lab to get the little cardboard kit and instructions.

When they return early the next morning for the second transfusion, Dr. Wilbur is there. He asks Dave what colour his stool samples are. Dave seems offended.

"What do you think I am, a dog? I don't look at my poop!" he says.

"We left the sample at home. Dave has one more to do. But what he's collected is kind of black," Pat pipes in.

"That could mean old blood," says Dr. Wilbur. "Pat, can you go home and get them and take them into the lab?"

Pat suggests perhaps Dave's esophageal ulcers have come back. He'd had that condition four years earlier.

"That could be it," replies Dr. Wilbur. "But you should get me the samples."

Pat leaves Dave at the hospital and whips home to get the stool samples. When she returns from the hour-long drive, Dave tells her he is scheduled for an endoscopy — a diagnostic test in which a small camera will be mounted on a tube and inserted into his digestive tract through his mouth — and that Dr. Umberto, one of their regular customers at Springhill, is going to do the procedure around about two o'clock that afternoon.

Later, the nurse comes for Dave. She wheels him away down the hall and Pat is left alone. She stares out the window at the brilliant blue sky and tries to suppress the concern that is rising in her mind. She calms herself by thinking it must be a reoccurrence of his esophageal ulcers. "He's going to be okay," she thinks to herself. "We're going to get through this."

Not 20 minutes later, the nurse comes back to get Pat. She is led into the examination room where Dave is lying on a gurney, wide awake but silent. Dr. Umberto, a slim man with a quiet, introverted manner, explains that they have given him a memory-blocking drug that keeps patients responsive but with no memory of the procedure. Pat recalls something about this drug from Dave's operation for an infected prostate.

She is standing beside Dave, holding his hand, when Dr. Umberto gives the results of the scoping.

"The news isn't good," he states baldly. "Dave has esophageal cancer."

Pat glances wildly at Dave but he just smiles back at her.

"Oh my God," she says, her voice barely a whisper. "But that can't be right! He hasn't complained of any pain," she manages to stammer inanely.

"That's the nasty thing about this type of cancer," the doctor says. "The esophagus has no nerves. It's just a hollow pipe. So it has no way to indicate when it is damaged or in trouble."

"Dave isn't taking this in," continues Dr. Umberto. "I know he looks like he's following what I'm saying but he won't remember any of it. You're going to have to tell him. But come with me for a minute, and I'll show you the pictures."

Pat follows Dr. Umberto to the little office around the corner and stands while he flicks the computer awake. "I took some great shots," he says, pointing at the screen. "Here's a really good one."

But then his words get garbled and Pat feels as though she is disappearing down a black hole. His voice is fuzzy, and she fights to focus on his words. She can't understand why he is so ecstatic about good photographs when he's just told her that Dave has cancer.

Pat takes a big breath and asks, "Is there anything that can be done? Can you operate?"

"That doesn't look like an option," says Dr. Umberto. "But we have to wait for the pathology report."

The doctor asks if Dave has been having any trouble swallowing.

"No," says Pat, "only with the large calcium pills, but he's eating everything just fine."

He tells her Dave will likely start to have trouble swallowing and that he will refer them to a cancer agency. He says they will know more once they have the pathology report but that will take a week or so to come. A nurse comes in. She hugs Pat, and leads her back to Dave, who has been moved back to the transfusion room. It will be another couple of hours before Dave will be able to fully comprehend information.

Pat sits down in the hard leather chair once more, gently takes her husband's hand and is glad that he is sleeping; for a little while longer he will be spared. It is the hardest two hours of her life, waiting for him to come back, dreading having to tell him.

* * * * *

It is in the car on the way home that Dave fully recovers from the memory-blocking medication. She has waited for him to ask if Dr. Umberto had said anything. Pat tells him that the doctor is pretty sure he has cancer, but that more tests have been ordered. She asks him to let her get them home before she fills him in with more details. He doesn't say anything. At a red light, she reaches for his hand, sees his eyes droop, his mouth turn, his shoulders sag. Dave's two brothers and his father had died of cancer. Mary, Springhill's farm market manager, had spent three years fighting it. All of them had lived with it for quite a while. "Sid," says Pat gently, "we can do this."

Pat watches Dave as he looks out the window seemingly oblivious to the little white church on Mission Hill, the summer flowers on the gravestones, the ripening fields of barley. As the scenery passes by, she steels herself for another battle. The cancer diagnosis isn't cause for despair. With all of Dave's health problems, they are used to fighting. She decides right then and there, they will get through this together.

But her resolve begins to diminish once they get home and start to research esophageal cancer on the Internet. That's when they realize how deadly it is, and how little it responds to regular cancer treatments like radiation and chemotherapy.

* * * * *

A few days after the diagnosis, they are driving home from an abdominal ultrasound appointment at the hospital when Pat decides to stop at Dr. Wilbur's office to see if Dave's recent blood work results are in. She wants to know whether Dave is going to need another blood transfusion this weekend. It is a quiet day and they get in to see the doctor quickly. Pat explains that they were just passing by on the way home from the hospital, from Dave's abdominal ultrasound, and they thought they should stop to see if the blood test results had come back.

Dr. Wilbur moves over to his computer and after a few keystrokes says that, indeed, all the latest test results are in — the blood work, the x-rays and the ultrasound.

"So fast?" Pat asks.

Dr. Wilbur doesn't look up from the screen. When he turns around, he looks solemn. "I'm really sorry, Dave," he says. "This isn't good news."

He explains that the x-ray and ultrasound tests show that the cancer has metastasized to Dave's liver and lungs. His words floor them. Until now, the cancer had been surreal. No symptoms. No pain. Just the endless, debilitating fatigue. But they know any additional threat to Dave's lungs is certain disaster. The spectre of Dave's breathing becoming even more difficult devastates them.

Dr. Wilbur's voice grinds on. He tells them to make another appointment in two weeks when the pathology report is sure to be back. "But I can't see that the report will change anything we already know," he adds.

He tells Dave he will set up an appointment for him at the cancer agency in Victoria. And he suggests that he get his affairs in order.

"How much time have I got?" asks Dave.

"It's always just an estimate," says Dr. Wilbur. "But I've seen lots of cancers. Your liver is very involved. So I would say six months is the most you can expect."

They stand up to leave and Pat isn't sure she or Dave will make it back to the car. He looks haunted and she feels weak and shaky. She takes Dave's hand and they walk out of the office. They are devastated. Dave's lungs are the weakest part of his body. He won't make it. In her heart, she knows they have already lost the battle, and they hadn't had a chance to fight.

Back at home, they hold each other, snuggled up into Dave's big leather recliner. They both cry, sobbing, their bodies wracked with grief. They stay wrapped in each others' arms for what feels like hours. Then Pat gets up and puts on the Tim Hortons coffee maker. Together, they sit down at the kitchen table overlooking the farm and decide to snap out of it.

CHAPTER 4
Cruising
AUGUST 2005

Minutes later, over coffee at the kitchen table, Dave and Pat decide to go to a party — on a houseboat in the B.C. Interior — a four-day celebration of a nephew's 30th birthday. They have been waffling on a decision for weeks, not sure Dave would be up to the rigours of summer road travel.

"Goddamit, Dave," says Pat, "who'd believe you'd have lung cancer on top of everything else?"

"Yeah, it looks like this is as good as it's going to get," says Dave. "If I've just got six months left to live, we better get some living in while the getting is good. Let's say to hell with it and just go, pull out this afternoon so we can be in Vancouver when Craig and those grandsons of ours come in from Australia."

"Great idea, babe!" Pat agrees. "I'll call Jackie and tell her we're in on the houseboat. Then I'll call Mom and Dad and ask if we can stay with them a couple of days, and I'll let Michele know we'll definitely be over." Most of their best plans have been made over coffee at their kitchen table and this was one of their easiest decisions.

Dave has another appointment with Dr. Wilbur in a week, to find out the results of the pathology report. In the meantime, Dave has no other medical commitments. He isn't feeling great — unusually tired — but he's always been up for traveling, and now there's more reason than ever to go. They both want to escape into the company of family. Forget about the cancer for a while.

Pat packs the clothes. Dave packs his meds. And that afternoon, Dave is behind the wheel cruising down the highway, heading for the tourist-packed, BC Ferries lineup. Despite his fatigue, Dave belts out, in a somewhat reedy voice, his traditional "cast-off" tune: Willie Nelson's "On The Road Again."

It has been many months since they last visited the girls and their families, in Australia. Michele, Craig and their two sons, Chris and Michael, now six and eight years old, have just moved back to Vancouver from Australia after five years living and working there. Both Michele and her sister, Lisa, have connections Down Under. Michele married an Australian physiotherapist, whom she met in Vancouver. Lisa moved to Australia in her 20s, also married an Australian, an agricultural scientist, and has never left.

Now that Michele has moved back, Pat and Dave spend the ride to Vancouver talking about how much their little grandsons will have grown. They can't wait to see them. There's so much to catch up on — their stories of packing up a household, saying goodbye, jetting first to Asia and then to Vancouver. Currently, Michele and her family are staying with friends until their own house is ready.

Every year, on the third Saturday of August, it is Michele's friends' custom to invite neighbours and work colleagues for a big backyard barbeque. This year, it has become a welcome-back-to-B.C. party for Michele and her boys. Pat and Dave had been invited and, at the last minute, they decide to accept the invitation.

At the party, they are surprised when introduced to a Dr. Vincent, a well-known Vancouver cancer specialist. The doctor's monk-like aura of calm seems disrupted, momentarily, upon meeting Dave and Pat. However, he smoothly acknowledges them and then turns to deal with one of his children. Although they hadn't actually connected with Dr. Vincent before this, Pat had been receiving his take on Dave's cancer, second-hand, via her old friend, Nurse Alexis. Pat had contacted her when

Dave's latest health crisis began. Alexis, with her cheerful, "fix-it" personality, had readily volunteered to ask a friend of hers, Dr. Vincent, for his opinion on Dave's test results.

Later in the evening, Pat notices Dr. Vincent attempting to strike up a conversation with Dave. But Dave doesn't seem up for the one-on-one socializing and drifts over to a group of people watching their host grill salmon on a cedar plank. It's a use of wood he isn't aware of. Alone with Pat later, Dave wistfully outlines possibilities for the millions of board feet standing on their forested 14-acre piece of Springhill. He already has so many ideas for what he could do with the land, but his ailing body won't let him.

The next day, after a five-hour drive up into the rolling hills of the British Columbia Interior, past lush orchards and vineyards and picturesque lakes, Pat and Dave pull into the parking lot of the houseboat rental company. They step out of the air-conditioned comfort of their SUV and into the blazing sun at the houseboat rental office.

This is their first visit to Shuswap Lake, the houseboat capital of Canada, and everyone is already there: Pat's sister Jackie, her husband, Lyle, and their sons, Ranger and Jason, with their girlfriends; Pat and Jackie's brother Dee; and three friends of the family. Blistering heat rises off the parking lot pavement and Pat feels perspiration already running down her spine. She looks out at the dozens of houseboats gliding on the lake and many dozens more tied up at the docks — floating RVs, huge, immaculate, two-level water homes with spacious decks, winding staircases, brass railings everywhere. Deluxe. Dave squeezes her hand, leads her over to the family group clustered under a scrawny shade tree. He grabs a chilled bottle of Corona from a cooler, flips it open and hands it to her.

Standing here now, surrounded by family, they're glad they made the trip. This is just what they need — a little time away from the misery of doctor's appointments and tests. A little time to enjoy the summer.

The lake is a deep, blue-green mirror, calm and glistening in the sun, the hills beyond a wooded patchwork. Their houseboat is still being set up: young men are running around shirtless, carrying boxes and luggage, gassing up the boat, giving cruising instructions to Lyle and Dave and the boys. Dave is fascinated by the mechanics of the boat and he listens avidly, asking questions about the steering and docking systems.

Pat notices the name of their boat: *No Bullshit*. She tugs Dave's sleeve and nods to the boat with her head. He smiles at Pat. "Well, that is just about all we can ask for in life, isn't it?"

Once on board, they're wowed by the setup. Three bedrooms, including one large bedroom on the main deck for Pat and Dave, complete with sliding glass doors and a private balcony. A kitchen with marble countertops and a dining room with wrap-around windows to enjoy the views. The men go up to the open-air top deck. Lyle claims the captain's chair, starts the engine and puts the boat into reverse. Soon they are cruising along the glassy lake, slipping over the cool, clear water.

Pat and Jackie go inside to make a pot of coffee and Dave comes down from the flying bridge on the top deck. He slides into the comfy banquette and starts tweaking his new camera, the one he got before his solo trip earlier in the year to Antarctica. Pat had refused to join him on that adventure. She didn't mind indulging Dave's obsession with travel. But she wasn't going to Antarctica. Months-long cruises were one thing; stormy seas with 25-foot waves were more than she was willing to contend with. So he went alone, with his camera, and came back with an elegant multi-strand necklace of freshwater black pearls from Buenos Aires, as well as an exquisite matching jewelry set of silver and black onyx. His photos had made her regret her decision. But his stories about being cinched down in his bunk to avoid being tossed about in the violent seas validated her original fears. He, however, can now say that he has walked on every continent.

Lyle stops the houseboat at a quiet place in the middle

of the lake and Ranger, Jason and their friends dive into the water. Pat goes outside with a cup of coffee for Dave and they sit together listening to their nephews' whoops of laughter, breathing in the warm air, redolent of baking hillsides and pine trees. Jackie and Lyle have arranged for a power boat with waterskiing equipment and two jet-skis to be delivered to the boat. Soon, plumes of water spray erupt from gunned engines and sleek boards. Dave goes into photographer mode.

Dave spends a lot of the day inside on his laptop — loading, editing, cropping his shots, getting organized to burn CDs for everyone to take home as a memento of this trip. When the sun begins to set, the men take up their positions on the top deck and psych themselves up to ram the boat onto a beach. They are to handle this floating hotel like a landing craft in a World War II epic. None of them has done anything like it before, and they are concerned that they'll rip the bottom out of their luxury barge. But the rules are that houseboats must be stationary for the night, so they have to trust the advice of the young men in the parking lot. Aiming the boat full throttle at the shore, they beach it easily. It works — simply and surprisingly smoothly. Brother Dee jumps off and drives a stake into the sand, tying the boat up to the stake with a rope.

Later, they all sit on the deck in the cooling air of evening and play poker under the stars. It is late, but the competitive tension is high. Nine defeated players, armed with beers, avidly follow the play of the last two combatants. Dave surveys the cards on the table, glances at the cards in his hand, looks up at Jason and says, "Well, kid, I've got you beat."

Dave casually pushes his stacks of plastic chips into the centre of the table. "Not only am I gonna call you, I'm gonna raise."

"I think you're bluffing," says Jason. "You don't scare me. I'm in."

And he promptly matches Dave's raise.

Dave slaps his cards onto the table. "Well, beat three kings," he says.

"With pleasure, man, I've got a straight!" Jason thumps down his winning hand for all to see.

Everyone guffaws and shouts. Dave shakes Jason's hand, his broad smile proof that for at least this brief time, the nagging knowledge of his impending death has disappeared into the background. Other than Pat and Jackie, no one else in the room knows about his cancer diagnosis.

Pat has been the dealer for this friendly poker game. She looks over at Dave as she packs up the cards and suddenly recalls one of their quick, mid-week getaways to Las Vegas.

"Hey, Dave," she says casually. "Remember the time we went to Vegas and you lost $250,000?"

Everyone's eyes light up. They sense a story. They all know that Dave is a bit of a VIP at Harrah's Casinos in Vegas and Reno, and that his passion, after family, farming and travel, is cards.

"I've never heard that story," says Jackie.

Pat lifts her eyebrows and smiles. "How about it, Dave, shall I rat you out?"

He nods sheepishly and grins; Dave is a man of few words.

"Well, we'd done our marathon drive down to Vegas," says Pat. "Twenty-two hours, pedal to the metal. Just stopping to potty our bodies, get gas and food. We'd switched off on the driving."

She tells them how Dave had gone straight to baccarat, his favourite game. And she went to play her favourite 25-cent slot machine — #5510. As usual, Dave played for hours on end. The pit bosses loved him because he bet nearly every hand and in so doing, kept the game going and the croupiers busy. Every few hours, she'd drag him away for a meal break — usually complimentary, thanks to the pit bosses. So this one night, Pat persuaded Dave to leave the game and join her for a beer and some nachos. They were sitting in the bar when she asked him why he didn't switch over to a different game, like blackjack. He said he was having a great time.

"Hmm. So what's a great time mean exactly?" Pat asked him. And then she voiced the awful thought that had just popped into her mind. "You didn't bet the farm, did you?"

"No," Dave grinned. "But I did have $250,000 go through my hands today."

Pat panicked. "God, Dave, what are you talking about? *Did* you bet the farm?"

"No, it's the casino's money," said Dave. "And I'm up! Just for fun, I thought I'd keep track. So for the last 10 hours, I've jotted down every play, added it all up and it comes to 250 thousand bucks that's passed through my hands. It's been a gas putting down the odd thousand-dollar bet. I figure why not — hey, it's their money."

She laughed. "You know, I thought you were playing a tad recklessly. I walked by your spot earlier when you had just put a hundred dollars on the tie. I didn't *say* anything. But I did *think* you were nuts! But then what do I know — you won! So I kept my mouth shut and left you alone to enjoy the crowd's appreciation of your nerve."

Pat winds up the storytelling saying, "You were ahead over $3,000 when you stopped that night, isn't that right, Dave?"

Dave nods, smiling. Pat looks over at him and thinks how much farming and gambling have in common. In both, there are so many unknowns, so little you can control. They have always been lucky in both.

Later, in the privacy of their bedroom, Dave feels free to release his repressed sadness and frustration. The warmth of the summer night thwarts their desire to stay locked in a lingering embrace, and inevitably the buildup of body heat forces them to separate. Most nights, their sleeping pills promote the blackness of sleep to block the dark forebodings that overwhelm them when the day's distractions cease. Dave remains his usual self — stoic, solid, dependable — in front of family and friends, but in the night stillness Pat feels him fall away from her, vanishing into his own worries.

* * * * *

Their first day back in Courtenay, Pat and Dave are back at the doctor's office.

"Your pathology report came back inconclusive," says Dr. Wilbur. "So we've sent it out again. We won't have the results for another week."

He continues his pitch to Dave about setting up oxygen at home, and then about making an appointment in Victoria, the closest big city, for an assessment at the cancer agency there. But Pat's mind is still stuck on the absent report.

"Can I see the reports for the ultrasound and the x-rays?" she asks, interrupting. She has no idea why she's asking. She probably won't understand them anyway.

Dr. Wilbur obligingly prints off the reports and passes them to her. She starts reading while Dave and the doctor finish their conversation. She sees the phrase "no pulmonary involvement" in the x-ray report. Her heart skips a beat. Wait, she thinks. Dr. Wilbur said the cancer had spread to Dave's lungs. His lungs, the weakest part of his body. He'd been dealing with COPD for more than 15 years and his strict adherence to a complicated regimen of medication is just barely keeping his breathing close to normal. If Dave did indeed have cancer in his lungs, his breathing would just get worse. Neither of them believed his lungs could cope with yet another deadly onslaught.

"Excuse me," she interrupts again, impatient. "This report says '*no* pulmonary involvement.'" She points to the words on the paper. "Does this mean Dave's lungs *aren't* affected?"

She passes the paper to the doctor. He glances at it.

"Oh, I must have been thinking about someone else," says Dr. Wilbur breezily.

"So the cancer hasn't spread to his lungs?" Pat asks, shocked.

"No," says the doctor simply, a response that strikes Pat as cavalier.

When they get up to leave, Pat can hardly contain herself.

As soon as they're out the door, she says, her voice laced with sarcasm: "Well, this is truly a Good Friday! You're cured of lung cancer!"

They leave Dr. Wilbur's office with a confirmed plan of action. The next week, they are to go to Victoria to meet with a radiologist and an oncologist. The cancer agency there will assess Dave and give him advice about treatment options and what to expect in the last few months of his life.

They decide to make their ritual stop at the local Tim Hortons on their way home. Dave orders his regular treats: a large double-double coffee and a Long John donut, no sprinkles. It's always the same. Pat gets herself an iced cappuccino made with chocolate milk. They sit down at one of the empty tables, nodding at some of the regulars.

"Don't you think it's weird that I asked to see those reports?" Pat asks Dave once they get sipping on their drinks. "I don't even know why I did that. It's not like I know how to interpret all that medical jargon. But then, the word 'pulmonary' just jumped out at me — Heaven knows that word has been said often enough in the last few years. But it took a bit for my head to absorb what 'no pulmonary involvement' meant."

"Well, it's good news, right? Just when we needed some," says Dave.

* * * * *

A week later, Pat and Dave head out to Victoria where Dave is scheduled for his first assessment at the BC Cancer Agency. They don't know what to expect from these meetings, other than what Dr. Wilbur has told them. Dave would find out exactly how the cancer will affect his body, all the horrible details of what will happen to him and what can be done to ease the projected onslaught of pain that is synonymous with late-stage cancer.

On the three-hour drive, Pat and Dave feel torn — they want to know what's going to happen, but they also don't want to know. Michele has offered to come along for support and they've gratefully accepted. As a nurse, she will be able to help them understand the medical details that go over their heads. Michele had come over to the Island a couple of days earlier with her husband and the grandkids. The little boys had never seen the new house, since Pat and Dave were still living in the old farmhouse the last time they'd visited.

The day before leaving for Victoria, Pat had taken the grandkids out blackberry picking at the Air Park. Pat and the grandkids take over the kitchen. Blackberries, tapioca and sugar are nestled in a deep baking dish between sheets of pastry. Chris crimps the edges and cuts the vent holes. Michael brushes the top with milk and sprinkles sugar. On the dinner table, their golden brown masterpiece with its hot rivulets of berry juice is the centre of attention, along with the tub of vanilla ice cream. Later, Dave trundles the little guys around the property in the small, orange utility trailer bolted onto the back of the ride-on lawn mower. Together, they cut down some clumps of Scotch broom and haul it all off to a burning pile — men's work. The boys love it, but Dave is more tired than ever.

Now, their two-car convoy winds its way into Victoria. When they get to the cancer agency, Michele accompanies her parents to their appointments. They are all stiff from the long ride, and from fear. They would all rather be with Craig and the boys driving off for a day of exploring B.C.'s capital city.

First, they meet with a radiologist who recommends radiotherapy, a kind of radiation, to cauterize the esophageal tumours in an attempt to reduce Dave's internal bleeding and possibly to reduce the size of the tumours. Dr. Richard, a small, harried man, launches into a rapid-fire description of the "palliative radiation" procedure. It's the first time they've heard that phrase. Pat asks for clarification and learns that it's radiation to offer comfort and pain relief to those who are dying. She hadn't thought radiation could offer either. But the doctor explains that because the esophagus has no nerves, pain relief/comfort would not be the object in this case. Instead, he says, the designation of "palliative" is an acknowledgement that this form of treatment can in no way be regarded as a cure for the cancer.

Another word — cauterize — worries them. Dave asks if radiation involves some sort of burning action, and the doctor admits that is exactly what radiation is, with ionized rays that are focused precisely on the body part that needs to be seared. Pat voices her concern that the esophagus is in close proximity to the lungs. She mentions that Dave's lungs are already severely compromised by COPD and asks if there is a possibility that the lungs could be burned during this procedure.

Pat's mind flashes back to a conversation a few years ago with Dave's lung specialist. She had questioned the constant heavy doses of prednisone being prescribed to Dave. She'd read that long-term use of prednisone was known to be extremely corrosive to all the organs of the body. The specialist had snapped back, "Nothing else matters if Dave isn't breathing!" Today, the radiologist is reassuring. He says it will be a low dose, and although there is no guarantee Dave's lungs won't be affected, the method of mapping the area being subjected to radiation is meticulously calculated. They will be careful.

Still, the information session with the radiologist leaves them feeling anxious and indecisive. It's been only a few days since they got Dave's lungs back, and they're just not up for doing anything that might cause harm to those already traumatized organs. A few minutes later, Dr. Stanley, a medical oncologist, enters the examining room. He has an easy, avuncular style, exuding a professionalism and warmth that immediately puts Dave, Pat and Michele at ease. After shaking Dave's hand, Dr. Stanley comments, "You're looking great! Much better than what I expected after reading your medical history." The elderly doctor asks Dave about the kind of farming he has done and about his travels, particularly Dave's recent trip to Antarctica. Eventually, the conversation turns to Dave's cancer. Dave wants to know if there is any possible way to beat the type of cancer that he has. The doctor explains, simply and honestly, that the options for dealing with esophageal cancer are very limited — high-risk surgery, chemotherapy and/or radiation — but that, in Dave's advanced case of cancer, it is far too late for any of these options to be effective. All Dave's other health issues, coupled with the fact that his cancer has already spread to his liver, means nothing would contain the disease.

"Indeed," stresses Dr. Stanley, "for you, chemotherapy would be a lot of pain for absolutely no gain." He says he has discussed Dave's case with Dr. Richard and that he supports the radiologist's call for low-dose radiation of the esophagus. Dr. Stanley encourages Dave to consider opting for Dr. Richard's services but fully understands the concern for possible damage occurring to Dave's lungs. Dr. Stanley says that minimizing internal blood loss will possibly reduce Dave's level of fatigue and help avoid the need for more blood transfusions. The doctor points out that too many blood transfusions can add unwanted problems to an already complicated situation.

"How long do you think Dave has?" asks Pat, blurting out the words. "Dr. Wilbur said six months."

"Could be," replies the doctor. "Could be three months. Or three years."

Pat and Dave exchange glances. Dave asks how the whole thing will play out.

The doctor asks Dave if he is having trouble swallowing. Dave replies that he has no symptoms other than fatigue. Incredible fatigue. Dr. Stanley expresses concern about Dave's future ability to eat. He says it's likely Dave will soon be in pain when swallowing, and will have difficulty eating. There will also be back pain from his liver. It will probably be excruciating.

"You know how these things are," the doctor says. "A crisis usually strikes when help is almost impossible to access — like at two o'clock in the morning. I want you prepared to deal with it promptly."

Pat asks if there is anything experimental that might be

available. Dr. Stanley says he is positive that there is nothing that can be done to avoid the inevitable. They are advised to just "go with the flow, and keep any pain in check." He says he will prescribe morphine and possibly OxyContin, that they should always keep these medications close at hand and that Dave should not hesitate to use them. Dr. Stanley also cautions them to refrain from mentioning, in public, the names of the drugs that Dave will have in the medicine cabinet. He says it is surprising how many times an overheard conversation is the impetus for drug addicts to target homes where strong pain-killing meds are in use.

"Dave, you'll probably sink into a coma before you die," says the doctor. "That's usually how it goes."

Listening to these words, Pat feels oddly detached. But her chest is tight and it feels as if the air has been sucked out of the room. She takes a deep breath and tries to focus on the information, on what she needs to know to be of help to Dave, on preparing herself for what lies ahead. She listens to Michele ask the doctor more questions, admiring her daughter's calm confidence. Pat turns to Dave, watches a storm of emotions pass silently across his face. She can see he wants to fight this. Despite the odds — despite his disappointment — he wants to tackle this. She can tell that Dave is appreciative of Dr. Stanley's straight talk. But for Dave, giving up is truly the last option. Then she recalls the specialist saying Dave could survive three years. Hope blanks out the bit about succumbing in three months.

* * * * *

Pat offers to drive home, but Dave assures her he would rather take the wheel. "It'll give me a chance to focus on something other than body parts and expiry dates," he says wryly. She wholeheartedly seconds the idea of a break from all the angst. He asks her to put on the radio to catch the traffic and travel report. Michele and her family are heading back to Vancouver, and he is concerned that the boys are going to be waiting for hours in a lineup on the ferry terminal's hot tarmac. When the announcer says there are no sailing delays, they turn the dial to find the news. It is so weird how the world can just keep going, when their own is imploding.

On the long drive back to Courtenay, Pat feels flat after such a long, emotional day. For Dave, though, concentrating on driving seems to be lifting some of the tension that he has been carrying.

When they reach Goldstream Provincial Park, their car shrinks in the shadow of the towering, 600-year-old Douglas firs and cedars. As the highway snakes through deep canyons, radio reception becomes annoying static.

"Can you turn that off until we get through here?" says Dave.

Pat has some CDs in the glove compartment and pops the top one into the player. It's Jackie's Christmas present to Dave, a selection of country music favourites that she downloaded for him. Dave and Pat belt out the chorus to Vaughn Monroe's "Ghost Riders in the Sky." They listen to Dave's favourite — Elvis's "Old Shep." When Kenny Roger's "The Gambler" comes on, they smile and start to sing along. Suddenly the key phrases become too personal, jarring.

You got to know when to hold 'em, know when to fold 'em,
Know when to walk away, know when to run,
'Cause every hand's a winner and every hand's a loser,
And the best that you can hope for is to die in your sleep.

They are simply unable to keep singing when the familiar refrain repeats.

Great tunes by Willie Nelson, Charley Pride and Waylon Jennings continue to fill the 4-Runner as it eats up the miles, enabling Dave and Pat to drift into a companionable silence.

With less than an hour left until they are home, Dave sets cruise control to 120 kilometres on the new stretch of highway above the retirement village of Parksville. Gazing out the window at the passing scenery, Pat is reminded of the drama that they'd lived through just 10 years before.

"Hey, Dave," she asks, "was it right about here where it all happened?"

He laughs, knowing exactly what she is referring to. "Close, we're coming up on it. Just there about a hundred yards before that next on-ramp, on the other side."

She and Dave were driving to Vancouver to pick up supplies for the farm. It was a cold, February morning and they were barreling along the deserted highway in their white, 16-foot cube van. They'd pulled out of Springhill at 4:30 that morning, giving them plenty of time to catch the first ferry at 6:30. Tiny snowflakes falling out of a dark, grey sky were beginning to settle on the blacktop. A small car whizzed past them. And then a lone tire raced by, making a single track in the fresh snow. She looked at Dave, to see if he'd seen it too. He had. They laughed and laughed.

"Wow," he said, "I wonder where that came from. It's a good thing that little car is long gone. That tire would do serious damage if it hit something that small."

But as soon as the words left his mouth, the van started listing to the driver's side. Dave began wrestling with the steering wheel and they could hear the awful grinding of metal on pavement.

Dave glanced in the rear-view mirror and yelled, "Damn. There's sparks right under the gas tank!"

He wrangled the van onto the gravel shoulder, the brake pads buried in stones. Pat used the cell phone to arrange to be towed into the GM dealership in Parksville, only to find out it would be impossible to get the van fixed that day. She remembers them scouring the bush beside the highway, battling the overgrown salal to find the tire. It had landed in the underbrush three-quarters of a mile from where the van had stopped. She remembers Dave's steely determination, straining every muscle as he managed to force the van off the highway. He has always been the strong one, literally steering them out of harm's way. She knows she could never have gotten that van safely off the road by herself. "God, how am I ever going to live without him," she thinks now to herself.

As they drive by the graveled lane leading to their old vegetable market, she tries to lighten the mood. "Man, we'd be picking corn right about now," she says, "and worrying about the pickle crop."

"And you'd be on the phone most of the night calling pickle customers to confirm their orders and which day they wanted to pick them up," Dave responds. "How the heck did we do all that?"

"I don't have a clue," says Pat. "I'm sure glad we're not doing it now."

"But you could've run the farm without me," says Dave.

"No way," counters Pat. "I wouldn't have wanted to. It was only fun with you."

CHAPTER 5
Settling
SEPTEMBER–OCTOBER

Pat couldn't have chosen a better day for a family reunion. It's a beautiful, sunny autumn afternoon and her entire family has gathered in the garden behind a picturesque, little white church in Richmond. Lisa had arrived earlier that day from Australia, heeding her friend's advice that she should be on the next plane. Her husband Michael, their twins, Matt and Nick, who are now five, and Vanessa, who is six, have come along as well. And now, all the little kids are running, weaving around the flower beds, while Pat walks with the photographer, organizing her 34 family members into small groups.

Pat has managed to pull off this huge photo shoot and party in just 10 days. This is the first time in five years that they have all been in the same place at the same time. And for the first time, great-grandparents Lewis and Christina van der Gracht will meet all five of their great-grandchildren together on Canadian soil.

With Lisa coming to town, and Michele having recently moved back, it seems the perfect opportunity for a family photo. Lisa's arrival coincides with Pat's birthday, as well as her sister Terry's birthday and their sister-in-law Valerie's. Pat had called everyone just a couple of weeks earlier to arrange everything. She told them, "Dave's really sick. We're not going to have a funeral. Both of us think that if people want to say something nice about another person, why wait for their funeral? It's better to say it to their face than to their coffin."

Dave was never aware the gathering was intended as a farewell tribute to him. He didn't know exactly what Pat had said when she phoned everyone up to invite them. He was just relieved she'd broken the news about his cancer to both sides of the family. He didn't have the energy, or the desire, to talk about it.

And yet, there is nothing maudlin about the afternoon. Everybody is looking forward to the party afterwards at Terry and John's place. Their son, Brian, is a chef and has flown in from Calgary to help prepare the food. Even in the frozen-smile moments of the photo shoot there is a sense of celebration — the happy chaos of a big family. Aunty "Shell" is reading books to Lisa's kids, letting her niece, Vanessa, try on her lip gloss. Dave is sitting and chatting with Lisa in the shade of the tall trees. He's all dressed up in a black shirt and blazer and he reaches out to pat the kids' heads as they run by. But to Lisa, her father looks haunted, morose — certainly not his usual self. She knows he doesn't want to be here, nor does she. No one likes getting their photos done, but they put on their best faces to make Pat happy. They smile, respond to polite questions and family conversations. Lisa talks about her husband's new job, her law studies, the plane ride from Australia.

No one talks about Dave's diagnosis. The unspoken tension is awkward, at least for Lisa, who can't wait to talk to her father — alone — about what is going on. She has only talked to him about it once, on the phone, when he had called to tell her he had cancer. Sitting here now with her father, she recalls that phone call one month earlier; how her first reaction had been devastation that her children would grow up without their grandfather, without his influence and love. "My kids won't get to know you," she had wailed, and then realized her own selfishness, focusing on her children when her father had just told her he was going to die. Hanging up the phone that day, she felt winded. And when she rushed off to pick up her kids from school, she told a friend, a doctor who knew all about esophageal cancer, about her dad. "How long do you think he has?" Lisa had asked. "Can I wait to visit until Christmas?"

"No, I wouldn't," replied her friend. "You should be on the next plane."

So here she is now, watching the photographer organize her extended family into small clusters. Then there is the final big shot: the whole branch of the van Waterschoot van der Gracht clan together. Everyone is poised, standing or sitting on the picnic bench under the large maple tree, the autumn sun dappling through the leaves. No one knows this will be their last hard-copy memory — of Dave, and of Pat's mother, Christina.

* * * * *

Back home in Courtenay, Lisa, Michael and their three children fill the house with laughter. Pat takes them out to pick the last of the blackberries along the walking trail at the Air Park. Dave is too tired to come along, though it is one of his favourite spots — the small planes taking off and landing, the view of the mountains and the expanse of the Courtenay River estuary ebbing and flowing along the wide pathways. He has been weak for some time now. To Lisa, it is shocking to see how much time her father spends in his recliner. She understood that his cancer caused fatigue but she hadn't realized the edema had so curtailed his mobility. The other day, when he'd switched his dress shoes for soft moccasins, she realized for the first time just how much his swollen feet were affecting his life.

She can see him reveling in the distraction her children provide — keeping them busy, playing cards and reading them books. But it is difficult for him to rest in the midst of so much childish glee. Michael helps Pat move another recliner into the master bedroom and shift the TV from the guest room so that he can get away from the family room whenever he needs to recover his strength. Once, when Pat goes in to turn on the TV, to block out the rising noise of the children, Dave gets angry.

"Turn that off," he orders.

"But it's getting so noisy out there," Pat replies. "I thought this would help."

"It's okay," says Dave, calming down. "I want to hear the kids. It isn't noise to me."

In the morning, Pat is reading to the children in the living room when Lisa walks through for breakfast. She sits down at the kitchen table in the alcove, beside Dave, and Pat can hear them admiring the giant maple tree. Its leaves are starting to change colour and the golden yellow is glorious against the bright, blue morning sky. They suddenly stop talking. Father and daughter look at each other. It's clear they are both thinking the same thing: that Dave won't be around to see the leaves next year.

That afternoon, Dr. Wilbur calls to ask if he can come by for a visit. He knows Lisa is in town because she had emailed him to ask for a letter to validate her absence from work in Australia. When he arrives, Dave's GP briskly asks to have a tour of the house. They're all surprised by his request, but to accommodate their guest, they comply. Michael takes the kids into the family room to watch a *Cinderella* DVD, closing the pocket doors to the formal living room behind him. The doctor walks through the house like a real estate agent, verbally approving of the large master bedroom, good-sized ensuite bathroom, well-appointed guest room, one level, no stairs — noting that these things will be perfect aids for someone dying at home. The four of them troop back to the living room and settle onto the sofas. But Dave remains standing. Dr. Wilbur dispassionately begins to talk about the process and the mechanics of dying at home.

"The first thing I'm going to need you to do, Dave, is to sign the Do Not Resuscitate order — a DNR. Having that on file makes things so much easier for us medical types. It means an ambulance doesn't need to be called, but if it is, the attendants are not obligated to do CPR. Plus, any doctor can come in, whenever they've got time, to pronounce your death. And, as I've said, we also need to get an oxygen condenser in here. I can get that paperwork started tomorrow and the machine should be in place by next week. Maybe set it up in that long hallway? They can attach plenty of tubing to reach your recliner in the family room and to get to your bed at the other end of the house. Putting it in the hallway will help cut down on the noise factor."

"I've already told you I don't want oxygen in the house," says Dave tersely.

"But the reason I gave you a six-month window," the doctor says, "is so you could qualify for in-home oxygen and community care."

Pat and Lisa are stunned. If that was indeed why the doctor had said Dave had only six months to live, then perhaps Dave actually had longer than that. Perhaps he *could* fight this.

Dave doesn't want to be here, doesn't want to talk about this. He just wants to be with his grandkids, not sitting around talking about cancer and oxygen and dying. Dave doesn't bother replying. He turns abruptly and stalks out of the room, joining the grandkids to watch their movie. Pat and Lisa look at each other with surprise, shrug and turn back to Dr. Wilbur.

Dave is not one to have his decisions contradicted. He does not want, or need, oxygen in the house and here is this doctor pushing it on him. Dr. Wilbur's intransigence triggers Pat's memory of another time when someone else had tried to do an end run around the Maddocks family.

Twin Hollies Farm had been sold to an investment consortium, but the Maddocks family had rented it back on a long-term lease. The family had then continued to maintain the large acreages of raspberries and strawberries. One spring day, Dave's brother Keith had phoned and informed Dave that this was the year that the lease was to be renewed, but the rent had sky-rocketed. Keith had found out that one of their competitors in the berry business had offered the consortium an outrageous rent to gain control of the soon-to-be-producing crops that the Maddocks had nurtured for the past many years.

Dave agreed with Keith that accepting the revised rental rate would be financial suicide. But they weren't willing to be ripped off like this. So, on the last day of the lease, Dave went over to Richmond, packing along his heavy-duty Stihl chainsaw. Keith was turning the strawberry plants into green mulch as his tractor and rototiller passed slowly over each row. Dave was felling the raspberry canes. As much as this went against everything they held sacred as farmers, they refused to be horn-swoggled.

When a cop car pulled up sometime later, an RCMP constable walked out to the field and interrupted Dave. The officer greeted Dave and asked him what he was doing.

Dave replied politely, "Pruning raspberries."

"So is this how raspberries are pruned?" countered the cop skeptically.

"Well, officer," Dave had drawled, "sometimes we prune them high and sometimes we prune them low. Today, we've decided on low."

The cop had smiled and returned to his car.

That left the consortium with no crops to harvest and, consequently, no tenants.

Dr. Wilbur's voice brings Pat back to her living room. He reiterates that if Dave is going to die at home, he needs to sign a DNR. "I can see Dave's not in the mood to talk about this. Are you sure Dave wants to die at home?" the doctor asks.

"We did talk about it," says Pat, "and he said he would prefer to be here rather than in a hospital."

"Well, make an appointment to come in and get the paperwork. I'll leave it up to you to get Dave to sign it. Are you okay with that?"

"Yes, I'm sure that will be fine; right now is just a poor time to have brought it up. But I am worried that I'm not capable of keeping Dave comfortable. I'm not sure I have the skills to recognize what will need to be done for him when things get really bad. The medical oncologist in Victoria said that Dave will probably slip into a coma and I just don't know how to deal with that."

"Pat, your job is to supply Dave with emotional support not physical care. We'll have nurses to do the physical part," he tells her. Then he adds, "Dave seems depressed."

"Uh, yes, he is," responds Pat. "But under the same circumstances, I think any sane person would be."

"Is he taking his anti-anxiety medication?" asks Dr. Wilbur.

"Yup. He calls them his happy pills," says Pat.

"You can tell Dave to double the dose."

* * * * *

A few days after Lisa's family leaves to go back to Australia, Pat and Dave drive to Port Alberni to visit Jackie and Lyle. Michele's husband and their grandsons will be there, too — Michele has to work. Jackie had bought them tickets to a local Sunday afternoon event called the Harry Potter Train and invited them all to sleep over.

The boys arrive in their costumes — with gnarly magic wands and black capes and star-encrusted wizard hats. After a dinner of barbequed salmon and Jackie's specialty, apple and rutabaga casserole, they play cards at the kitchen table until late. Dave is happy to be there, enjoying the games of Happy Suitcase and War with his grandsons around the kitchen table and chatting with Lyle. But his edema is worsening. His feet are swollen; the skin stretched painfully, marginally relieved by frequent massages with a foot salve. He can only manage to walk short distances. Dave has his feet up, but he doesn't like sitting for so long. That position makes breathing more difficult.

Dave's abdomen has become so enlarged that he can no longer wear jeans. Only extra-large sweatpants are comfortable. Being divested of the uniform of a farmer is a sad blow. He wants to go out and walk the old farmstead with Lyle, package spuds, schmooze with the grocery store produce guys. But he is too exhausted.

At 1:00 a.m., Pat is woken by the phone ringing. She knows it can't be good news. Through the bedroom wall, she can hear Jackie talking. Pat gets up, careful not to wake Dave, and knocks quietly on her sister's bedroom door.

"Is everything okay, Jackie?" she whispers.

Jackie comes out and they go downstairs to the kitchen together.

She tells Pat it was their sister Terry who had phoned to say their mother had just gone into surgery at Vancouver General. They were hoping to repair a burst aortic aneurysm. This wasn't supposed to happen. Their mom was diagnosed with the aneurysm last December but her cardiologist vetoed the surgery for many reasons: she was 84, overweight, sedentary because of arthritis, and she has a history of severe heart disease. They were all told that when the aneurysm broke, she would die instantly. But, it seems, the last layer of skin had held.

Now, these new doctors offered her surgery, saying she would have about a 10 percent chance of surviving. They warned her about the high probability that the surgery would cause a heart attack, but she said yes anyway. Terry had reported that as they wheeled Mom into surgery, her last words were, "Don't let them cremate me!"

Jackie and Pat know they must go to be with her and to help out their dad. They plan to catch the first ferry off the Island.

Pat doesn't want to leave Dave, but he will be with Craig and Lyle, whom she knows Dave can rely on. She wakes Dave just before 5:00 a.m. to let him know what has happened. She crawls into the warm bed beside him and tells him quietly why she has to leave. She promises to be back in time to drive him to his first radiation treatment at the cancer agency in Victoria on Monday. Dave and Pat's mom have been great gambling buddies over the years. He is upset to hear the awful news about Christina, but agrees that he just could not deal with the stress of a fast trip to Vancouver and the quick turnaround to get back to Victoria. Even half-asleep, Dave is valiant and assures her he will be just fine.

It is still dark when she and Jackie head out to the highway. When they arrive at the hospital, they are so thankful for what VGH has provided for their family. They have a large, private room with several chairs, a couch and a recliner. Their father, three brothers, other sister and their families are all there. Their mother is in the intensive critical care unit, in a one-bed, glass-walled cubicle down the hall. They take turns going in to be with her, usually in pairs.

Christina had indeed had a massive heart attack on the operating table. Her body temperature had plummeted so low that the surgeons were forced to stop the operation. They were unable to close the huge incision. With tubes coming out of every possible orifice, Mom's every bodily function is being controlled by machines. She has a nurse devoted to her care exclusively, 24/7. Their regal "Queen Mum" looks like a creature from *Star Wars*.

It's Pat and Jackie's turn to visit her. As each of them gently holds one of her hands, Pat listens as Jackie asks for an update from the nurse. Jackie has been an operating room nurse so she fully understands the information. There is mention of rising creatinine levels. Pat senses that she needs to know the significance of this. She asks the nurse to explain and the nurse draws Pat over to a corner of the cubicle.

"The creatinine level gives us a good indication of the health of the kidneys, and if they are still able to perform the critical job of flushing toxins out of the body," she says. "Your mother's level is hovering around the 250 mark, which is worrying. We are doing everything we can to avoid going over 300, which would mean the kidneys are in extreme danger of failing completely. If that happens, your mom would need dialysis, probably every day for the rest of her life."

Pat manages to thank the nurse. But she is confused and upset. Getting her mom through her heart attack a few years ago had been scary. This complication is mind boggling. The nurse rechecks the readings on a couple of machines and then carefully begins to massage Mom's feet with lotion. Pat is awed by the nurse's compassionate, thoughtful gesture.

"Everyone is here for you, Mom," Pat whispers gently in her Mom's ear. "Everyone is praying for you. Dave is rooting for you too, and sends his love."

Her mom's lips and jaw begin to flex and quiver.

"Please don't try to talk, sweetie," Pat pleads. "You have a tube in your throat. Just move your head a tiny bit, if you can. Are you trying to tell us something? Are you thirsty?"

When she nods yes, Jackie passes Pat a package containing a small, moist sponge. Pat quietly informs her mom that because of the tube in her throat, she is not allowed to drink. Her mother gives a soft mewling sound. She opens her eyes and they are frantic. Pat quickly tells her that she is getting lots of fluid intravenously.

"Mom, I can moisten your lips and the inside of your mouth with a damp sponge. It has a minty taste. Do you want me to do that?"

She gives a little nod, and Pat carefully swishes the damp sponge over her Mom's parched mouth.

Several times that day, Pat and each of her family members have the opportunity to spend a few minutes by their mother's bedside. But she becomes less and less responsive. Though the cubicle is spotless, the linens pristine, the hum of the machines muted, the attendants dedicated, Pat feels like her mother is imprisoned in a nightmarish, futuristic torture chamber.

Pat can't understand why her mother would have made this choice. Her mother was almost crippled by arthritis, and yet staunchly refused the use of a wheelchair. She was in agony from the pain, but she would not allow morphine to pass her lips. Her mother was a fervent and devoted Catholic, and yet, when push came to shove, she chose to cling to this terrible existence.

Oddly, it reminds her of the cabbage plant. Pat had harvested heads of cabbage thousands of times. Dave didn't work up the fields after taking off the crop, as the root mat developed by all the plants would help prevent the erosion of the soil by winter rains. But a couple of weeks later, little green buds would have formed around the edge of the cut cabbage stem. Six weeks after that, perfect baseball-sized heads of cabbage would be thriving. Lop off those little heads and the stalk would try, yet again, to grow. Only the blades of the rototiller going through the field in the spring would end the plants' efforts.

Life needs to *be*. It craves existence. It has absolutely nothing to do with reason or logic. It is totally divorced from such abstracts as intelligence or philosophy. Although disturbed and dismayed by such determination, Pat finds it impossible not to deeply grieve its defeat. She straightens her shoulders and looks around the room. Surrounded by family and nurses, she is grateful for all the care and attention bestowed upon her mother.

Pat knows she will have to leave the next day. Take the two-hour ferry back to the Island, drive two hours to pick up Dave, still in Port Alberni, and then, the next day, drive another three hours to Victoria where he is scheduled to receive his first of four doses of radiation. She says goodbye to her mother, and that familiar feeling arises again — she doesn't want to leave. She feels pulled, twisted and torn, like a kite caught in a tree.

* * * * *

The night before they are set to drive to Victoria for Dave's first radiation appointment, Pat can't sleep. She is lying beside Dave in bed, feeling the heat of his legs beside hers. She wants to rest her head on his chest, but that only makes his breathing more difficult. He takes her hand and she feels herself dissolve. The tears fall. She can't help herself.

"What am I going to do without you?" she sobs, knowing her question is unfair.

"Don't worry, Pat," he says, gently, reassuringly. "I'll be with you. Always."

She tries to push her overwhelming sadness away, to cherish this moment, lying close beside the love of her life.

She is grateful now that her mother's history of illness had long ago prompted Pat and Dave to create their will, decide on cremation rather than burial, determine where to spread the ashes. They don't have to talk about any of that. They don't have to talk at all. She knows Dave prefers it that way. She closes her eyes and focuses on the warmth of her hand in his, and their sleeping pills slowly take effect.

* * * * *

On the drive to Victoria the next morning, they barely talk. Neither of them knows whether radiation is the right thing to do. They are so worried about the possibility of lung damage, but the doctors all seem to think it is a risk worth taking to stem the blood loss from his esophageal cancer lesions. They aren't so sure. His breathing is more laboured than usual and Pat can hear him wheezing in the quiet of their SUV. She can't imagine it getting any worse. They are worried, too, about radiation sickness, although the doctor has assured them the dosage is low.

It is now early October. It has been almost two months since they were last here. Dr. Richard, the radiologist, seems put out that they have taken so long to decide. Pat again explains their concern about Dave's lungs; how they weren't sure he could handle more damage to that part of his body. Dr. Richard says he understands, that he will make the markings very carefully. True to his word, the doctor spends well over an hour marking Dave's body, leaving little dots all over his chest.

The treatment itself takes only a few minutes. And when they return to their room at the BC Cancer Lodge, Dave seems more depressed than usual. He passes the time playing blackjack and solitaire on his laptop. The next day, they return for a second round. This time, the whole process only takes a few minutes.

Back in their room once again, Pat suggests they go to visit her aunt and uncle who live nearby. But Dave says no, he doesn't want to do that. Pat persists. "But it's a perfect opportunity, Sid. Let's get out of here."

"I can't do that," says Dave, weakly. And he starts to cry.

His tears astonish her. He has only ever cried in front of her once before. They had just bought the farm in Port Alberni. Pat had stayed behind in Richmond so that Michele, then in kindergarten, could finish school. Dave was living on his own in the little, green farmhouse, cooking and cleaning for himself, marketing the remaining storage potatoes, learning the ins and outs of this new farm and getting their first crop of spuds — 125 acres of them — planted and growing.

Every other weekend, Pat would visit with the girls. One Sunday, when she was packing up the kids and the car to go back to Richmond, Dave came up behind her and gave her a big hug. He hung on to her, not wanting to let go. She felt the sobs before she saw the tears, his sturdy body shaking against hers.

"Sweetie, what's wrong?" she remembers asking.

"It's just that I really miss you guys," he said, tears coursing down his handsome face.

Pat recalls feeling completely surprised. For him, she thought this temporary arrangement was a big, exciting adventure — striking out on his own to start up another farm. Until that moment, she hadn't known how much he needed her. All through their lives together, Dave has given her so many lovely things. But that simple, heartwrenching declaration of his love for her and their girls remained, always, the very best gift she had ever received.

Today, the tears are different. They shock her into realizing how desperately ill he really is and how powerless she is to ease his turmoil. Years ago, she had calmed him with her assurances that, within just a couple of months, they would be together again. Now, as she holds him, they weep together. This time such promises are impossible.

After two more radiation sessions, Pat and Dave drive home. In the car, Pat realizes the radiation has had an unexpected side effect. Dave didn't get sick. He got sad. Nothing she says, not music, not even silence, can break his melancholy.

The latest update on Pat's mother has increased their anxiety. The day before, the surgeons had taken her back into the operating room to close the incision. The threat of infection had become critical. Since returning to the ICU, Pat's mom had shown no signs of awareness at all. That Dave is too weak to be there for her has made him more downcast than ever. Dave insists that Pat leave him at home and return to Vancouver herself. He is adamant that he can fend for himself and promises her that he will call Phil, their basement-suite tenant, if he needs help.

"I am so sorry I can't come with you to see your mom," he says.

"Please don't worry, Sid," she replies. "Everyone totally understands. Mom knows you love her. But, of course, I'll tell her again."

They pass the rest of the ride staring out the windows.

CHAPTER SIX

Introductions

SEPTEMBER–NOVEMBER

Back in early September, when Pat and Dave are in Richmond visiting Pat's parents and celebrating their grandson's birthday, Dave is relaxing, flipping through a newspaper. At home, they'd never bother getting the Vancouver editions, but coffee and reading the big city newspapers are a pleasant morning ritual here.

Dave's eye is caught by "Promising New Drug Targets Prostate Cancer" in bold black print. He reads the lengthy article that features several quotes from Dr. Vincent, the Vancouver oncologist they met at Michele's friends' barbeque. Apparently, an organic protein is being used to surround and smother a cancer mass rather than the traditional chemotherapy method of infusing the entire body with powerful poisons to kill the rogue cells. The news piece forecasts a brilliant future for this revolutionary molecular anti-cancer process that incorporates an individual patient's genetic material.

Dave hands Pat the section, pointing out the article he's just read and commenting that he hadn't known that Dr. Vincent was such a big bug in cancer research. Pat scans it. "It's too bad that this new approach seems to be focused entirely on prostate cancer," she observes. "But hey, who knew we were hobnobbing, again, with a celebrity! Remember, there was the political party president who bought your watering system; then that TV news anchor we met at Club Med in Cancun; and the former B.C. premier on that flight to Narita and then he introduced us to Canada's ambassador to Japan when we were all waiting to grab our bags off the luggage carousel. Hmm, I really don't think we can count the two Playboy bunnies on the flight to Sapporo who showed us their write-up in the Playboy newsletter to prove they really were who they said they were. So now, with Dr. Vincent, that makes five newsworthy types we've been associated with. Too cool!"

"Hold on! I'm adding us to that list!" Dave objects with a grin. "Both you and I have been quoted, *with pictures*, at least five times in the Courtenay papers. And you made it into that 'around-the-city' column in Italy. Remember, when you fainted and fell backwards into that glass display case in Venice and split the back of your head open on the stone floor. They even had a picture of that ambulance powerboat whisking 'the English lady' away."

Dave and Pat share a chuckle.

That evening, Pat phones her friend Nurse Alexis. They had planned to meet for coffee the next day but Dave wants to head for home first thing in the morning. Pat mentions seeing the newspaper article quoting Alexis' friend Dr. Vincent. In chatting, Pat comments that they hadn't known Dr. Vincent was so involved in cancer research, that his work sounds really promising and that it's too bad the focus is on prostate cancer, not on esophageal and liver cancer. Alexis says that she, too, had seen the story and was intrigued by how much less toxic this new approach to cancer treatment seems than what is currently in use.

There is a lengthy pause and then her friend says, "Pat, could you put Dave on the phone? I'd like to talk to him."

Pat turns the cordless phone over to Dave. He is on the phone a long time. Alexis is doing most of the talking. Eventually, Dave says good night and hangs up.

Pat is curious. "What was that all about?" she asks.

Dave tells her about their conversation. "Well, you know

Alexis has been asking Dr. Vincent's opinion on my test results and what the doctors have been telling us. So he knows that I've been given six months to live. Alexis says Dr. Vincent actually tried to talk to me at the party about the possibility of me volunteering for a clinical trial." He pauses. "You know, I had a feeling he was trying to corner me for a private chat, but I just wasn't up for it. Anyway, later, Dr. Vincent asked her to talk to me about it, but she decided not to. You remember she did three years nursing at Children's Hospital, in oncology ..."

Pat nods.

"Alexis said that what those kids go through in clinical trials is heartbreaking and, almost always, it does them no good at all," he continues. "But that piece in the newspaper today seemed to be talking about a treatment with a radically new approach that maybe isn't poisonous like everything else that is being tested. So, I told her to tell Dr. Vincent that I'd be interested in finding out more about this trial idea. She said she'll get back to us."

Absolutely nothing had changed. And yet that night they go to bed feeling lighter than they have in several weeks.

A couple of weeks after they return home, they get an email from Alexis. In it, she says that Dr. Vincent isn't comfortable having Dave as his patient because of the friendships involved. So instead, he gives Alexis the contact details for the secretary of another researcher, a Dr. Xavier. Although they don't know anything about Dr. Xavier, they figure they can trust a referral given by a friend of a friend.

Right away, Pat follows up.

"We understand from Dr. Vincent that you are looking for clinical trial volunteers," Pat writes in an email. "My husband, Dave Maddocks, would be interested in finding out more about it. Dave is currently considering having four sessions of low-dose radiation that were recommended to possibly cauterize and maybe shrink the tumours in his esophagus. Would that disqualify him from being considered for a clinical trial?"

Dr. Xavier calls the next day. With a precise European accent, he tells Pat there is no hurry for them to meet as it takes four weeks for a clinical trial to receive approval, and four weeks is also the period of time that must elapse between radiation treatment and initiating the clinical trial. Dr. Xavier says having the radiation treatment done in Victoria is perfectly fine. They schedule an appointment with this doctor, in Vancouver, on the afternoon of October 21st.

In the meantime, there is so much to occupy their time. The definitive pathology report still hasn't arrived. The last one suggested Dave's esophagus wasn't the initial cancer site. Additional blood tests are done and Dave is scheduled for even more blood transfusions. But in the back of their minds, there is the ever-so-faint hope that there is something experimental and cutting-edge that will come to Dave's rescue. A possible course of action to follow where now there is none. At the very least, it seems worthy of exploration. It seems to give Dave a new spark, a reason to get out of bed in the morning.

* * * * *

It turns out the appointment with Dr. Xavier, is on the same day, Friday, October 21, as the funeral rites for Pat's mother.

After Dave's round of radiation treatments that Saturday, Pat had dropped him off at home and then hurried over to Vancouver, so she was at the hospital for the family conference her mom's doctor had requested. All Pat's siblings and her 87-year-old father were there when the doctor told them Christina's chances of survival had shrunk to less than 5 percent, that her kidneys had completely failed and that she had been in a deep coma for a few days. He recommended that the life support machines be turned off. The grieving family unanimously agreed, and within 27 minutes of disconnecting the machines, Pat's mother died. She had been hanging on by a mere thread.

The morning of Dave's scheduled meeting at the Vancouver cancer agency, they attend the funeral service in Richmond.

In the afternoon, Pat misses the internment to take Dave to his appointment, accompanied by Michele. Pat doesn't mind missing the burial. They have always been hard for her. When Pat was 10 years old, a little brother died and her grief-stricken mother had jumped into the baby's grave trying to retrieve him. Pat could never shake that image. Dave's appointment provides her with a way out.

Pat, Dave and Michele arrive at the cancer agency in their formal, funeral clothes: Dave in his charcoal-grey suit and tie, Pat in her fitted black dress. They enter the building, an eight-storey facility beside Vancouver General, through the sliding glass doors, past people waiting and reading in chairs, down corridors, up the elevator. The agency is packed with people. At the admitting desk, they are told Dr. Xavier is busy. But a Dr. Quentin, a resident oncologist, will see them shortly.

The three are ushered into a stark examination room. No one has explained why they are seeing a resident. Michele and Pat aren't impressed and they give each other looks of concern. Dave seems as tired as ever and disinterested. Dr. Quentin enters the room; he is curt and clinical and, without much explanation, performs a 30-minute head-to-toe physical, with Michele and Pat right there in the room. That too seems odd. Then he says he is going to get Dr. Xavier. Eventually, Dr. Quentin ushers in Dr. Xavier, with whom Dave and Pat have had only email and telephone contact.

Dr. Xavier, a tall, slim young man with an aristocratic air, says he thinks it might be possible for Dave to have chemotherapy. Pat tells him they have heard otherwise from Dr. Stanley at the cancer agency in Victoria, that Dr. Stanley said it would be "a lot of pain for no gain." But Dr. Xavier insists there are benefits to chemo at this point in Dave's disease.

Dave and Pat are courteous and continue listening. But they know from previous ultrasounds that Dave's liver is irreparably damaged; they have seen those pictures. They mentally discount the doctor's efforts to have them reconsider chemotherapy. As a farmer handling livestock, Dave is fully aware of how even healthy livers are not capable of coping with the onslaught of proven poisons.

Eventually, Dave interrupts: "What about a clinical trial?" That is, after all, what they are here to investigate. Dr. Xavier says the only one available is a Phase I clinical trial of a drug called CPX-1. He explains that CPX-1 is a combination of two common chemotherapy drugs — Irinotecan and Floxuridine — both well known and successful in treating cancer, but now combined with a fat liposome for a new kind of intensified, consistent treatment.

"Oh my God!" Pat and Michele say in unison. They hadn't realized the only trial being offered was chemotherapy-based. They thought they had come to talk about genetic, molecular trials, the next wave of cancer treatment. But apparently there isn't one of those trials currently available. CPX-1 is it. Michele and Pat are immediately defensive, protective. They don't want this for Dave. They've all seen, first-hand, the disastrous side effects of chemotherapy. But Dave asks the doctor to tell them more.

Dr. Xavier says that the clinical trial sponsor is recruiting for the sixth group of three or four volunteers, or cohort, of a proposed eight cohort study. He goes on to say that five cohorts are currently receiving CPX-1 infusions but all of them are at lower doses than the dose amount scheduled for the sixth cohort. Dave asks what the test results have been for the fifth cohort. Dr. Xavier explains that volunteers are given an MRI only after every two cycles, or four weeks, and a scan hasn't been done yet of the members of the fifth cohort. But, he adds, a woman in the fourth group had an MRI done after eight weeks on CPX-1, which showed her tumour had shrunk. Dr. Xavier leaves that piece of information hanging in the air.

Hope. It is like a beacon in a sea of despair and exhaustion. It has already been a long day, but Pat begins to feel a ray of light seeping through the fog in her head. She listens more intently now, as Dr. Xavier explains the rules.

If Dave is accepted, they will have to move to Vancouver for the first 30 days of Dave's participation in the trial. They can't stay with Pat's dad in Richmond, as they would normally do, but must find accommodations close to the agency — at their own expense. After taking the drug, Dave must present himself for 16 blood tests at specific times over five days; being close to the lab is mandatory since delays in traffic might upset the strict timetable. Dr. Xavier explains there are a number of tests required from Dave before he can be considered for the trial — blood tests, ultrasounds, EKGs, CT scans. His body has to meet certain standards. He has to have adequate function of his heart, bone marrow, kidneys and liver to metabolize the test drug. Pat perks up when she hears this. She knows Dave's lungs and his heart have been giving him serious health problems for many years. And his liver is in terrible shape. He's not likely to qualify. But she doesn't say anything. She's watching Dave to see what he wants.

Dr. Xavier says they can get started with those preliminary tests today, right now. Dave nods his consent. Pat can't believe it. She wants time to think.

Dr. Xavier explains further that if Dave is accepted into the trial, he can go home after the first 30 days, as long as they return every two weeks for another infusion. Pat asks if they can go cruising during the period of time between infusions.

"Or we could do a cruise after," suggests Dave.

"Good idea," says the lanky researcher. "I'd love to go on a cruise," he adds wistfully.

"Well, that's perfect," offers Dave. "You can come along and take care of me. We'll just put you in our suitcase."

"But would Dave be well enough?" asks Pat.

"Could be," the doctor responds.

"Sid," Pat says turning to Dave, insistent, "Why don't we go on a cruise *before* you do this?"

Dave looks at Pat then, frowning. He knows what her question means. They have an agreement. Pat will only go on one cruise per year. If Dave had his way, he'd be cruising and traveling year-round. Pat, on the other hand, wants time at home, to enjoy their house on the hill, to wake up to their fabulous view, and not have a farm to run. This year, they have already been on a lengthy European cruise. Her question — why don't we go on a cruise? — has a secret meaning just for Dave. He knows with those words that she doesn't want him to do this.

Dr. Xavier's optimism, this discussion of future plans, of vacations yet to take, bolsters their flagging spirits. When Pat looks over at Dave, he is smiling. And yet, Pat can't help but think about Mary, their robust former farmstand manager. They had watched her disintegrate with chemotherapy, lose her hair, her strength. Dave had built a ramp to her front door so she could easily get into her house in her wheelchair.

Pat feels herself flipping from hope to despair, as fast as if she were a fish on a dock, struggling to get back into the water. She is terrified of chemotherapy, but intrigued by this new information, about the possibility of Dave's recovery.

"Is what we're talking about here palliative chemotherapy?" asks Pat, trying to absorb all this new medical information. She had been reading about using chemotherapy for comfort and care, despite its horrid side effects. What Dr. Xavier was saying didn't jive with what they'd heard in Victoria from Dr. Stanley, whose words "a lot of pain for no gain" kept going through her head.

"No," Dr. Xavier replies, then quickly adds, "What do you think it is?"

"Well," she says hesitantly, "that we're going for the gold ..."

"Exactly," responds the doctor.

Michele is sitting on a black stool by the door, with warning signals going off in her brain. Dr. Xavier had mentioned earlier that they would transfuse if Dave's hemoglobin went below 90. In her experience that wasn't true. She starts to wonder about the doctor's expertise. "How long have you been in cancer research?" she asks when there's a break in the conversation.

When he says two years, she realizes that they aren't dealing with an experienced researcher and resolves to try to talk her dad out of this. The fact that Dr. Xavier hadn't personally given her father the hands-on physical was also making her uncomfortable. Her father's belly had swollen considerably since she had last seen him and he was sleeping in his recliner most of the day. Obviously, his tumours were growing quickly. But Dr. Xavier hadn't said anything about that.

Michele, who had been holding back throughout the meeting, suddenly interrupts, "You know, my father was diagnosed with terminal cancer and we were told by Dr. Stanley at BCCA in Victoria that he might not live past Christmas."

"Well, those predictions aren't always accurate," says Dr. Xavier.

Michele knows he is right, of course. No one can predict exactly when life will end. But she also considers her father's condition is far too advanced to handle chemotherapy.

"I *will* have to think about this," Dave says to the doctor. "But seeing as how I'm here, I'll do the preliminary tests to see if I'll qualify."

With that, they leave the office and head upstairs for blood work. The wheels are set in motion.

* * * * *

Michele returns with her parents to Courtenay for a few days to help them sort through the information and make a decision. She wants her father to understand his options. She sits with him in the kitchen, the table covered with papers — research documents and articles — and she explains the side effects of chemotherapy. She wants to articulate clearly the probable nausea, diarrhea and pain that will result from this chemotherapy trial. She wants him to understand that he could make a different choice. He could die quietly and peacefully at home, with nurses coming in to make sure he's comfortable.

She reviews all the wonderful things he has done to build up the farm and she encourages him to consider this option. "This would be a beautiful place to slip into a coma, Dad."

But he doesn't want that. He says he wants to make a difference.

Michele presses him. "Well, you can certainly fight with all you've got, Dad," she says. "Go for the research trial realizing you can die in the process, or you can have a peaceful death at home."

Dave replies quietly, "Michele, the truth is, whichever route I take, I'm going to die."

Dave is adamant now. "I don't want to slip away peacefully," he insists, choking back his emotions. "I want to *do* something. If this trial can do some good for someone else, then that's reason enough for me to sign on. I would rather die *doing* something *useful*, something for the future, than fade away hunkered down in this house."

Overhearing the conversation, Pat knows she will have to respect Dave's decision, whatever it is going to be. But she has a growing sense of unease about Dr. Xavier. He hadn't gotten to know Dave like Dr. Stanley had. Dr. Xavier hadn't personally given Dave a thorough physical examination; he'd only looked at Dave, whose outward appearance always belies the medical mess that his insides are in. He'd even recommended traditional chemotherapy when Dr. Stanley had said, categorically, that route would be pointless.

"You don't have to do this, Dave," says Pat.

"Dad, please," adds Michele. "Let's think about this."

"But the drugs being tested in this trial *are* well known," says Dave. "Doctors have been dealing with them for years. One they've been using successfully for 30 years and another for 9 years. So they know how to manage them."

"But, Dad," she pleads, "chemotherapy is poison."

Both Pat and Michele are torn between their own desire for

a painless death for the man they love, and the need to respect his wishes. They stay awake talking until the wee hours of the morning. Michele tells Pat that usually it is the white blood cell count that is decimated with chemotherapy and that would leave her dad susceptible to germs, and that the fast-approaching flu season would make things worse. Dave has long ago fallen asleep. He seems to be sleeping all the time now. They are both relieved he doesn't yet have the pain normally associated with late-stage liver cancer, nor the difficulty swallowing or eating that is normally associated with esophageal cancer. He's just tired ... and slowly slipping away.

* * * * *

Dave, Pat and Michele visit Dr. Wilbur's office the next day to go over the DNR forms. But Dave refuses to go in and stays in the waiting room. He doesn't want to talk about dying with anyone but his closest family. Michele tells Dr. Wilbur that her dad is investigating the possibility of joining a Phase I clinical trial in Vancouver.

"What!" exclaims the doctor.

"Some doctors at the BC Cancer Agency suggested my dad might be eligible for a chemotherapy-based trial, and Mom and I are both very worried about it," says Michele. "Dad's so sick. What do you think?"

Dr. Wilbur says Phase I clinical trials are extremely risky. Michele asks him if he can check it out for them, and he agrees. She offers to give him Dr. Xavier's number.

Two days later, Dr. Wilbur phones. He tells Pat he's had a lengthy conversation with Dr. Xavier and is very impressed. As much as he is against the idea of Dave being in a Phase I clinical trial, he got the feeling Dr. Xavier and his team are a caring group.

Disappointment. Pat was hoping Dr. Wilbur would say, unequivocally, after getting further information: "Dave, don't do this!" She wanted Dr. Wilbur to return with fact-based advice that would convince Dave not to do the trial. Until now, the arguments around whether or not to do the trial have been coloured with emotional concern. Pat and her girls do not want him to suffer. They want, desperately, to shield him from anything that could make his dire situation worse.

* * * * *

In early November, a fax comes from the BC Cancer Agency. Their office machine spits out the Subject Information and Consent Form, all 14 pages of details and ground rules for the trial, its risks and conditions. Pat shouts its arrival to Dave, who is in his recliner watching the ducks on the reservoir.

"I don't need to read that," he says.

Pat walks over to him from the front office. "You have to sign it. So you need to read it."

"No," he says. "I can make up my mind without that."

"Well, I'm going to read it to you then," she says. "You have to know what's in it."

Dave is frowning, pissed off that she is being so insistent. But she drags the leather ottoman over to his recliner and sits down beside him to read aloud.

"You are being asked to take part in this research study," she begins. Her throat suddenly constricts, then she starts again. "You are being asked to take part in this research study because you have an advanced cancer and your cancer has grown or spread after treatment with standard therapies. It is not yet known if the drug being evaluated in this study, CPX-1, will be able to kill cancer cells in people."

She goes on: "This is a Phase I clinical trial. Phase I clinical trials are the first studies of a potential new treatment in humans. In these studies, researchers evaluate how a new drug should be given (for example, by mouth, injected into the blood or otherwise), how often and what dose is safe. Because less is known about the possible risks and benefits in Phase I, these studies usually only include a limited number of subjects who have not been helped by other known treatments."

The document explains that the purpose of the study is

to determine what dosages of a new drug can be safely given to subjects with cancer. "Subjects are given the drug and monitored very closely to see what side effects they have and to make sure the side effects are not severe."

Pat takes a deep breath. She must stop herself from crying. The two of them have a pact. When they have something important to say to one another, she is *not* allowed to cry. He's always said it wasn't fair. Because he loves her, he wants to comfort her if she's crying. In those circumstances, he could never make a rational decision. So she holds back the tears. Her throat is sore, her voice cracking, as she keeps reading.

"Your safety is our primary concern. And your study treatment will be discontinued if you experience severe side effects ... Subjects will be given CPX-1 and will be watched closely to see what side effects may develop and to make sure that if side effects are seen, they can be taken care of rapidly.

"However, since there is very little information about the drug's effect on cancer in humans, we do not expect that you will benefit from taking part in this study, although the knowledge gained may benefit others.

"You do not waive any of your legal rights ..."

She gets to the end of the document and looks up at Dave. He looks indifferent, like he's far away.

"Well," she says, "at least they'll look after you. It says that Imodium is the main remedy. Hey, that's a staple in our travel kit. And it says they are willing to be held legally accountable. That's *got* to be good. And it says they can be inspected by Health Canada and even the US Federal Drug Administration." Pat pauses. "Sid, you know this whole thing scares the hell out of me but it is your decision to make."

He says nothing.

Pat goes back to the office to play Scrabble against the computer. Dave turns on the TV. They are both in their own worlds, each seeking distraction from a cruel reality. If he opts for the trial, he will be putting poison into his frail, deteriorating body, but by doing so he might be helping in the fight against cancer. If he opts to stay home, he will avoid the upheaval and possible dreadful side effects but continue to feel useless. Either way, he will probably only live a few more months. Neither option looks good.

Later that night, Dave comes into the office where Pat is zoned out playing Scrabble. He's in his heavy terrycloth bathrobe, with its muted green and purple stripes, a gift from Michele.

"I'm going to bed," he says.

Pat swivels around in her office chair and puts her hands under his robe to hug him. Her arms reach around him and she lays her head on his naked swollen belly.

"I'll be right in," she says, holding him.

"Pat, I won't do this trial if you don't want me to," he says. "But, you know, *I* want to do it."

Pat swallows. "It's okay, Sid. If that's what you want, that's what we'll do."

The decision is made. Pat is relieved. She doesn't have to think about it anymore. Dave has asked for her support and she is going to give it wholeheartedly, even though she doesn't agree.

CHAPTER SEVEN

Testing

NOVEMBER

The days before they are scheduled to return to Vancouver for the final tests to determine whether Dave will qualify for the trial, Pat is busy packing up their clothes, enough for 30 plus days away from home, readying Dave's oxygen machine and walker, checking ferry schedules and making meals. Dave is organizing his myriad of medications into a suitcase. He has so many pills for so many different things that he has to take at various times of the day: Vasotec, Pariet, pravastatin, Didrocal, prednisone, zopiclone, puffers and nebules of Pulmicort, Ventolin, Oxeze, Atrovent, plus the prescribed creams, eye-drops and tablets he uses "as needed" and the bevy of cancer related remedies he has recently been prescribed. A full-size carry-on suitcase would be his make-shift medicine cabinet. The nebulizer machine that allows Dave to inhale medications contained in the plastic nebules would have to travel separately.

Dave's pharmaceutical regimen is complex, but he has it down to an artful science. Too weak and his edema too pronounced to do much walking, Dave concentrates on this one task of organizing and packing up enough medications for a month. The cancer agency faxes through an extensive schedule of lab tests and test drug infusions that Dave will be expected to keep, appointments up to mid-January of the coming year. The two weeks to determination day, D-day, drag, and yet speed by. Pat finalizes the details for their accommodations during the month-plus period when they will have to be in Vancouver for the preliminary tests and the first portion of the trial — if Dave gets in. She reserves a room at the Vancouver Cancer Lodge with twin beds and a private bathroom. She's glad the room rate is so reasonable — about a hundred dollars a day — including meals provided by the in-house cafeteria. There is a nurse on-site around the clock, and the Lodge's nurse manager assures Pat they can provide a recliner for Dave; she doesn't have to worry about renting or buying one. The whole setup is such a relief. They would otherwise have had to rent a room in a downtown hotel.

When she slows down for even a minute, Pat is awed that their lives could be more intense than even the past few months. Because of the trial, there is suddenly so much to do. With Dave too ill to help, Pat has become the facilitator, preparing their lives for this trial. In the duet of their marriage, it's not a role she's used to: Dave has always been the one to make things work smoothly, more enjoyably — from the Rubbermaid turntables he purchased to help Pat and her crew when creating thousands of hanging flower baskets every spring, to sharpening the knives before she went out harvesting broccoli, to collecting mini-pussy-willow bouquets, her favourite, along the ditches of their farm.

One thing currently crystallizes the undercurrent of despair that permeates their every waking moment — Springhill's irrigation system. Pat has asked Dave several times in the last couple of months to show her how to deal with the irrigation system that Dave had installed in the front lawns. She needs to know how it works — how to schedule it, how to program it, how to shut it down and winterize it, how to start it up in the spring. The control box is an electronic nightmare to her: a 16-station commercial unit originally used to activate the almost hourly feedings of an acre of hydroponic greenhouse crops. The user manual was lost ages ago. The information is all in Dave's head. Each time she has asked him to show her, he has put her off. This morning, looking out over the lawns and evergreen trees coated in a thick layer of hoarfrost, she realizes her need to know is urgent.

Dave has such confidence in her ability to improvise, to pull off seemingly impossible tasks. So as not to add to the demoralizing and lengthy list of things now impossible for him to do, she has worked hard, especially over the past few months, to mask her dread of life without him. But her ineptitude with technology undermines her resolve. Now, sitting on the floor by his recliner after their morning wrestling match with his elastic stockings, she looks up at him with pleading eyes.

"Sid, please, can we look at the irrigation setup for the lawns today? There could be a really hard frost while we are away and all the pipes could burst. You know I'd do it myself, but I don't have a clue about what has to be done. Just tell me what you need and I'll gather the stuff up."

Pat doesn't want to disturb him. He can't afford to lose any strength if he's going to be able to do this trial, and showing her will take massive effort. But she has to ask. It is the only moment left. It is freezing outside and she knows the poly pipes will break. It's not important for Dave anymore; he's focused on living. But Pat is trying to be efficient and look after things.

She can tell he isn't up to it, but he asks her to get the wheelbarrow out of the garage along with plastic bags, long twist-ties and the multi-head screwdriver. Slowly he gets up out of his recliner and slips on his moccasins, shuffles his swollen feet outside. He unscrews the six C-clamps so that all the water lines can drain, then instructs Pat to cover the ends of the pipes with plastic and to secure each one with twist-ties so that insects don't move in. He pulls the electrical plug out of the wall, gets Pat to lift the control box off the support post and place it in the wheelbarrow. With the wheelbarrow back in the garage, he plugs the control box back in and shows Pat how to remove the backup battery. He is so beat. Pat decides not to push for a reprogramming demonstration.

The lesson is done with few words, both of them understanding the implications of this transfer of tasks. They don't talk about what Pat will do when she's all alone in this big house on the hill. Talking isn't Dave's style. But sadness, regret and love are in his eyes.

* * * * *

They arrive at the Vancouver Cancer Lodge in the afternoon of a cold, grey November day. The building is hidden behind tall, bare trees lining the street. The Lodge is conveniently located just a block away from the cancer agency where Dave will have all his appointments, tests and CPX-1 infusions — if he is accepted into the trial.

Inside, the Lodge is airy and bright, with a vase of fresh flowers on the reception desk. There's a common room just off the main lobby with big, comfy chairs, an aquarium and a piano. They are invited into a small office for intake. After the usual pleasantries, the nurse asks Dave about his cancer and the details of the Phase I trial. She then shows them to their room, just down the hall from the lobby. The room is small, but there is enough space to maneuver the walker around the beds and into the wide doorway of the bathroom. Basic, functional — Motel 6.

The nurse comes by a while later to see how they are settling in. Dave is already ensconced in the recliner and expresses his heartfelt gratitude that the Lodge was able to supply one. Pat asks if there is a TV available, but the nurse informs her that it is the Lodge's policy to only have TV available in the common areas, that the management wants to encourage residents to interact and be sociable. It's the same policy for Internet accessibility and food. Everything is available in the main common rooms. The nurse offers to show them the amenities, but Dave doesn't have the energy. He tells Pat to go off and tour the building herself.

The next day, they spend hours at the cancer agency. Dave gets blood tests and is asked to fill out several less-than-sensitively phrased survey sheets with questions about his sex life and his thoughts on dying. Then he has to swallow what seems like a gallon of an unpleasant, faux-orange concoction before going into a chamber to hold his breath — no small feat for someone with chronic obstructive pulmonary disease. Dave has been fasting all day, and the orange liquid will dye his esophageal tract so the doctors can see his cancer more clearly on the CT scan.

When they return to the Lodge after all these tests, Dave is tired and sinks gratefully into the recliner, dozing fitfully for the rest of the afternoon. Pat takes out a book, but can't concentrate on a single word. She pulls out her knitting and gets to work on yet another stretchy toque for the grandkids. She keeps messing up though, and has to rip it apart and start again, over and over. She is anxious about whether Dave will be accepted into the trial. She so hopes he will be, for that is what he wants and it would be unthinkably cruel to undermine, in any way, the huge effort he is making to achieve that goal. He wants to do the trial so badly.

She takes the elevator upstairs to the second floor cafeteria where she gets Dave some dinner — soup and a roll. From the line-up, she looks out the big windows at the bare trees being whipped by the wind trapped in the towering concrete-and-glass canyon that dwarfs the Lodge. The cafeteria, with its oil paintings of bright flowers and with fresh carnations on every table, is a cheery antidote to the bleak view. Pat thinks about their home back in Courtenay, already decorated for Christmas, and is relieved that they managed to get that done before they left.

If Dave is accepted, they will only have this weekend to go back home before returning to Vancouver again for an entire month. That would mean they wouldn't be back home again until December 21, at the earliest. Too little time to organize Christmas; Pat had realized that if she didn't decorate in advance, it would never get done. And the house is going to be full for

Christmas: Lisa will be coming from Australia with her husband and the kiddies, and Michele will be there too with her family.

Pat and Dave had set up the Christmas tree, reminiscing as the seasonal family treasures were dug out from their wrappings of year-old newspapers: the little waxen angel with the green, velvet gown and golden wings that they had bought the first Christmas after being married. Again, the ornament stood guard atop the rough cedar crèche that Dave had hammered together almost 40 years ago. The black papier-mâché donkey, one of Michele's elementary school projects, nestled in the skiff of hay, next to the manger waiting for the Baby Jesus figurine to magically appear on Christmas Eve. They took out the varnished and intricately carved Dutch wooden cows that Pat's grandmother had bequeathed to them knowing Dave had managed Twin Hollies' dairy herd. And crowning the tinseled, twinkling tree was the caroling angel that Lisa had crafted in art class out of a *Reader's Digest* magazine. And so many little decorations, handmade by their young grandchildren.

They'd discussed and bought gifts for all the grandchildren, squirreling them away, to be wrapped closer to Christmas. Pat arranged to have a metallic, cherry-red scooter delivered after they return home — her gift for Dave. And for the coming weekend, if Dave feels well enough to go home, Pat has organized a small birthday party for him with a few friends. Lisa is arriving from Australia in time for the celebration, coming alone for just one week to spend some quality time with her dad. She will return again with her whole family for Christmas, but she wants to be there for his birthday. He is turning 69.

Pat carries Dave's dinner down to their room, passing the activity room with its racks of newspapers, board games, half-finished jigsaw puzzles and blaring TV. Later, both craving a cup of coffee, she persuades Dave to get up and they walk down the hall to the activity room. He sits at the table, surrounded by other cancer patients, watching the news. The sky has long turned dark. Bowls of fresh fruit on the table remain untouched, but the evening tray of sandwiches is eagerly being snatched up. Some patients shuffle in and out, some in their bathrobes, opening the fridge at the back of the room for a drink or a snack, something to fill the hole of nausea, hunger and anxiety.

The next morning, they spend more time at the lab and then back to the Lodge for lunch. They return to the cancer agency in the afternoon to meet with Dr. Xavier, to get the results of Dave's tests and find out whether Dave has been accepted. When they get there, they meet Nurse Betsy, who has until now been only a soft, bird-like voice on the phone. A tiny young woman, she greets Dave and Pat with a fleeting smile and apologizes that Dr. Xavier isn't available today, that a Dr. Timothy is filling in. As she leads them down a labyrinth of hallways, Nurse Betsy raves about the professional expertise of Dr. Vincent, whom they'd met at the barbeque, and this new specialist, Dr. Timothy.

In an austere examining room with blue and yellow walls, Dr. Timothy introduces himself to Dave and Pat. He reminds Pat of every substitute teacher she ever had in school: competent but not engaged with the people in the room. He tells Dave he has been accepted into the trial and brings out a slew of papers — the Subject Information and Consent Form. Dr. Timothy asks if they have read everything. It's all business. Dr. Timothy requests Dave's signature and he signs on the "subject" line, legal proof that he is fully informed and consents to be injected with the experimental cocktail CPX-1. Dr. Timothy then asks Pat to sign as witness, and then Dr. Timothy adds his signature. Nurse Betsy leaves to make copies of the documents for Dave. Dr. Timothy tells them that Nurse Betsy is their liaison with the researchers; that they are to contact her with any concerns and to report any side effects as itemized in the consent form. When Nurse Betsy returns, she writes the after-hours contact phone number at the top of Dave's copy. The doctor gives Dave a prescription for an anti-nausea drug that he is to take prior to coming into the agency for the infusion on Monday morning. In less than half an hour, the contract has been sealed. And yet, there's no champagne. No balloons. No "atta-boy." No "thanks for this." It's completely anticlimactic.

They return to the Lodge. Dave is totally pumped at his being accepted and wants to head home straight away for the weekend. He asks Pat if she can get packed up quickly, travel now rather than the next day. She is more than willing to oblige. They have only been away from Courtenay for a couple of days, but it feels like a year. They don't care if they have to wait several hours for a ferry to the Island. They just want to go home.

Late that night, snuggled down in their own bed, they realize that they have missed the physical comfort of being in the same bed together. It is a relief to have the din of the city, the seemingly endless wail of sirens, replaced by peace and quiet.

* * * * *

Lisa arrives on her own by plane the morning of Dave's birthday, just in time to head out to the Japanese restaurant for the surprise lunch party Pat has planned. Dave *is* surprised and pleased to see the small gaggle of his closest friends, already there. Pat had deliberately invited people from all parts of his life: from his youth, from his farming days, from his life now — Dave's childhood buddy and best man, Harry; his nephew Lyle, who worked with Dave at Twin Hollies Farm in Richmond and at Port Potato Farm in Port Alberni; Larry, who had been Dave's right-hand man on Springhill for years; and Phil, their long-time tenant. Of course, their ladies were to accompany them. Pat hadn't been sure this party would happen. She didn't think Dave would want to come home for just three days before the first infusion. But she's glad they made the trip home, thrilled she could offer this small party to her husband.

Over bento boxes, they reminisce and laugh. Dave seems happier and more relaxed than he has been in months. Pat watches him eat his tempura prawns with gusto, listens to the easy conversation between him and his friends and family.

There is no dwelling on cancer or cancer trials. It is, Pat thinks, just as she had envisioned — a less boisterous version of an Irish wake but with "the dearly departed" present. The "eulogies" are fun and Dave gets to hear them, to join in, to reminisce about some of the moments that shaped his life.

"Remember when you took your 4-H group to the dairy calf competition at the PNE?" asks Harry. "You loaned your car to that kid. He returned the keys but forgot to tell you where he parked the car. How many acres did you cover that night looking for it, Dave?"

Dave laughs.

"Remember the time you got food poisoning while we were camping with my kids at that remote lake in the Cariboo?" adds Harry. "You thought you were done for. Remember, you'd just started going out with Pat. You wrote that 'it was great to know you' note and made me go to town to mail it."

Lyle interjects: "Remember that time you fell in the ditch when a bunch of us were out deer hunting in Port Alberni? Almost up to your neck in water and the only thing we worried about was the cigarettes getting wet!"

Then he adds: "Remember the time you were riding your Suzuki over those mountains of wood chips that we had stored up for that drainage project? You flipped the bike and it landed on top of you and broke your leg. But you passed out, so the damn thing burned your leg as well. That was really bad timing, Dave. You were in a cast for the whole planting season. That thing really itched, eh, Dave?"

Larry, their former Springhill field manager, pipes up: "Remember the time you were remodeling the ceiling of the potato pit with a chainsaw and it bucked back and sliced down behind your ear? Were you surprised that your baseball cap didn't stop the blade? What was that, Dave? Seventeen staples and two stitches in the lining of your brain and you didn't even have a headache!"

It is a really nice 69th birthday party!

Lisa and her dad spend the rest of the day hanging out together in the living room while Pat finalizes what she needs to bring along that she hasn't already left at the Lodge for the upcoming 30-day vigil. The next day they are leaving again, for Vancouver.

In the morning, Phil comes up from his basement suite to say goodbye and wish them luck. He offers them two eagle feathers, bound with bright blue cord intertwined with beads. One feather is bigger than the other, but both are beautiful, majestic.

"The bigger one represents you," Phil says to Dave. "And this one is you, Pat. I'm giving these to you as a blessing on your journey. That all should go well."

When they walk out the door to their SUV, the cold winter air is refreshing and clean. The house is decorated for Christmas. The beds are made, anticipating the influx of all nine members of their family. The car is packed — walker, oxygen condenser, suitcases, pillows. Lisa is with her dad. They are ready.

* * * * *

When they arrive at the Lodge later that night, Dave eagerly heads for the recliner, exhausted from the long trip. Lisa heads off to stay with friends. In the morning, they head up to the Cancer Agency for his first dose of CPX-1. Dave walks slowly in his soft moccasins, pushing his walker up the sidewalk. It's a bright, sunny day, but the late November wind is cold.

They proceed through the automated front door of the agency, and take the elevator to the sixth floor. A very pregnant and jovial nurse escorts them into a room. She is chatting about her upcoming maternity leave as she settles Dave into one of two big, green leather chairs and inserts the IV needle into his arm. The experimental chemotherapy drip is going to take 90 minutes.

The nurse sends Pat down to the in-house pharmacy to

have them fill a prescription for Imodium. She wants them to have it on hand just in case Dave experiences diarrhea, which is listed in the consent form as a 50-percent-possible side effect of CPX-1. The nurse stays in the room with Dave, monitoring his vitals and, every 30 minutes, taking a blood sample. Every 30 minutes, a young woman carrying a small, insulated cooler shows up to collect it. Pat notices her efficiency and precision and is comforted by her appearing on the dot at exactly the right time. Dave is going to have to get used to all these blood tests. He has agreed to give 16 more over the next five days. They will be walking over to the cancer agency's lab from the Lodge, sometimes more than once a day.

Dave watches the nurse who is busy charting entries into a log sheet.

"That's beginning to look like the reams of planting record logs we used to keep," Pat says. To help pass the time, she tells the nurse about Dave's work.

As they had farmed 36 different vegetable crops, keeping detailed records was essential. Every two weeks, they would sow an eighth of an acre of radish seed and then all the other acres of crops that went in as the soil warmed up — peas, potatoes, fava beans, corn, to name just a few. As well, they'd had 14 plantings of various transplanted crops every year. If Dave hadn't diligently kept track, Springhill would have been a disaster. Farming, says Pat, is all about observation and timing. If you don't stay focused on the health of your plants, you don't get a profitable result. Farming is science, just like this.

Together, Pat and Dave look out the window at the city: False Creek down below, the bridge humming with traffic, the mountains in the distance. Pat remembers how meticulously Dave would document the amount of fertilizer he would use, the date he seeded, the date he used herbicide, the date he sprayed for maggots, the date he irrigated, the dated harvested. Now, it is Dave's health that is on the line and he needs at least the same amount of careful monitoring and timely intervention, if not more.

As the nurse siphons off another blood sample, the collection gal with the insulated carry case enters the room. Dave and Pat are reassured. They are expecting this kind of attention to detail — after all, this is a scientific experiment — and today, those expectations have been met. After the IV bag empties, they leave the building, feeling confident that Dave has made the right choice.

* * * * *

That night, their room at the Lodge is crowded with family. Lisa, Michele and her family, and Pat's father, Lewis, have come to visit. The little boys begin a game of tag and the level of conversation is getting loud. To escape the craziness, Pat suggests they all move out into one of the common areas where they'll have more space to sit and talk. Their family takes over most of the lounge. Every chair is occupied, and others squeeze together onto the big comfy couches. The coffee tables are arranged with fresh flower arrangements. There is a fire crackling in the fireplace. The kids are watching the fish in the aquarium. With the piano and the book-lined shelves, the room is so warm and cozy; it could be someone's living room. Lisa is relieved to see that her father seems fine. "I'm glad you survived, Dad," she jokes. She had been worried about her father all day. Her Aunt Terry, Pat's youngest sister, had told her it's a good sign if you can get through the first day of chemo.

There are a few other people from the Lodge in the lounge as well. A man who volunteers at the Lodge to host singalongs comes in with a guitar. He sits down and starts taking requests. Lewis suggests "Danny Boy," his wife's favourite song. As the man strums the tune, the rest of the family joins in:

Oh Danny boy, the pipes, the pipes are calling
From glen to glen, and down the mountain side ...

The song's sorrowful lyrics about parting and loss slowly fill the room as more people join in. Abruptly, Dave gets up with his walker and pushes it down the hall to the activity room. Pat can see him chatting to a couple they had met earlier who were interested in Dave's drip irrigation system. Her family is singing, tears trickling down their cheeks. Pat decides to leave the party too and join Dave. She is so glad Dave has managed to escape this maudlin moment. She appreciates that her father is grieving the loss of her mom but Pat is annoyed that he has inflicted his pain on this place that is so full of its own sad stories. As she walks towards her husband, she can hear the closing refrain:

... You'll come and find the place where I am lying
And kneel and say an "Ave" there for me.

With a few deep breaths, she is able to hang on to her resolve not to be downcast — especially when the day has gone so well. She comes up beside Dave, loops her arm with his and joins the conversation about watering systems and plants. It is a great alternative to the display of heartache down the hall.

* * * * *

Early on Day 2 of the trial, Dave experiences three bouts of diarrhea. Consulting the consent form, Pat immediately gets Dave started on Imodium. He is to take two pills initially, and then one pill every two hours until he is clear of the problem for 12 hours in a row. Dave is not thrilled to be taking yet another medication, and so frequently. When he hasn't had a reccurrence for several hours and balks at taking more pills, Pat begins a record log. She keeps track of when he has diarrhea and the time he takes the Imodium. That way she can just show him the record and he doesn't give her grief about taking so many pills, so often.

The first few days pass slowly and uneventfully. Their routine quickly becomes predictable and tedious. Pat and Dave make the regular morning trips up to the cancer agency lab for his blood work. And every time, the collection gal has been there, on time. The weather has turned much colder and the sidewalks are slippery. The rock salt remedy is hard for Dave's moccasined feet, even with the help of his walker.

Most of their time is spent in their room at the Lodge, reading, sometimes talking or playing games on their laptops. Lisa has returned to Australia, and Michele, who has come down with pneumonia, isn't visiting until she's better. It's flu season, and other visitors are staying away to reduce the chance of an infection that could compromise Dave's already weak immune system. Three times a day, Dave and Pat go up to the cafeteria for meals, but the building is so full of patients that Dave rarely wants to go to the common rooms for a change of scenery.

To keep at least some semblance of normality in their lives, Pat walks the six blocks along Broadway to the closest Tim Hortons to pick up their regular afternoon indulgence. It is too far for Dave to walk. Pat has been checking out the many pharmacies and medical aids stores in the area trying to find a solution to ease the elastic stockings on over Dave's terribly puffy feet, ankles and now legs. They tried baby powder, but the perfume was too irritating for Dave's lungs. She had been unsuccessful in trying to find pure talc. Then, at one shop, she discovered a contraption called Easy Slide Caran, made from parachute cloth. They'd ordered it for her, and she was picking it up today.

That morning — Friday, Day 5 of the trial — Pat had contacted Nurse Betsy for advice. Just as Dave had feared, the Imodium has bunged up his system and he hasn't had a bowel movement for three days. The trial nurse told her to get Dave started on a stool softener, Novo-Docusate, that could be purchased at any drug store. So, Pat picks that up, along with the parachute cloth contraption and their Tim Hortons goodies.

The next morning, Day 6, Pat goes to help Dave put on his pressure socks using their new Easy Slide Caran. Having read the elaborate instructions, she is psyched up to give it a try. But when she goes to wrap it around Dave's leg, she is shocked to discover his swelling has completely disappeared. The edema in his feet, ankles and legs is gone. He needs neither the gizmo, nor the stockings. They are both ecstatic.

For the past few weeks, Dave hasn't been able to wear shoes at all. Now, suddenly, he can wear them again, but Pat hadn't brought any of his regular footwear with them. Buoyed and relieved, Dave asks Pat to go shopping for him — for shoes *and* a TV for their room.

She returns a couple of hours later with new shoes and slippers, two warm shirts and a small, portable TV set. Pat clambers over the recliner, anchoring the antenna so it is hanging out the partially open window. Dave calls out when she finally gets it positioned effectively. They watch the evening news together that night, laughing and joking. It is pleasant, comfortable and easy — a return to normal.

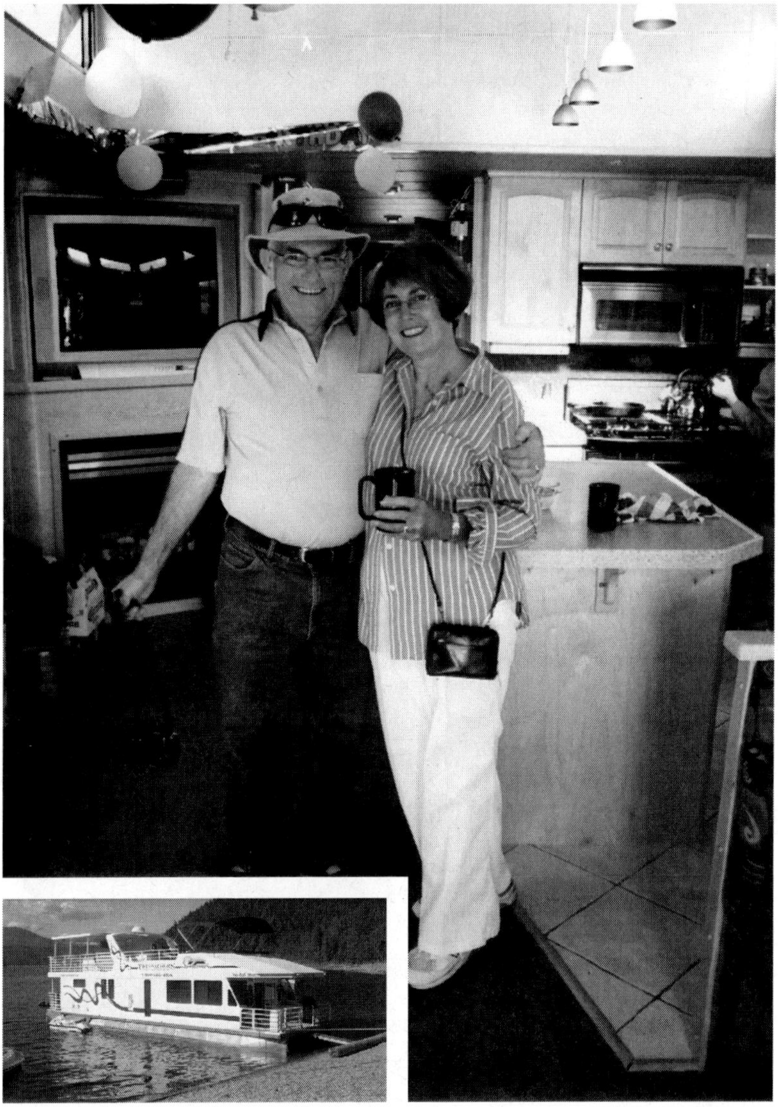

Pat and Dave in the galley of the houseboat Pat's sister Jackie rented to celebrate her son's 30th birthday. The deluxe craft on Shuswap Lake (see inset) was a "huge, immaculate, two-level water home with spacious decks, winding staircases and brass railings everywhere." This particular houseboat had been christened *No Bull Ship*, a play on words that prompted a smile from Dave and the response, "Well, that is just about all we can ask for in life, isn't it?"

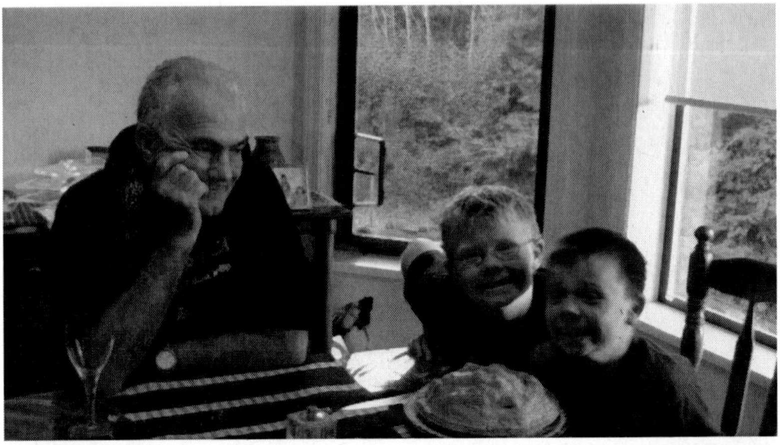

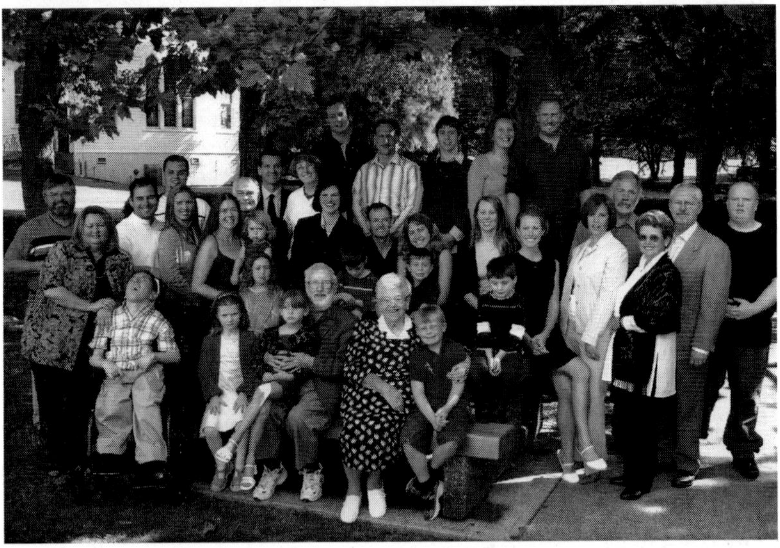

Top: Dave with his grandsons, Chris and Michael, as they are about to dig into a blackberry pie that the boys made with Pat, August 2005. **Bottom:** On September 25, 2005, the van der Gracht clan gathered to celebrate the return of Dave and Pat's daughters and their families from Australia. It coincided with the birthdays of three van der Gracht ladies: Pat, her sister, Terry, and Pat's sister-in-law, Val. **Opposite page:** The man who walked on every continent: Earlier in 2005 Dave went on a solo trip to Antarctica. For Pat, vacation cruises were one thing, stormy seas with 25-foot waves another. So he decided to go alone. His later stories about being cinched down in his bunk to avoid being tossed about in the violent seas validated Pat's original hesitation. On his return, Dave presented Pat with an elegant multi-strand necklace of freshwater black pearls he found in Buenos Aires.

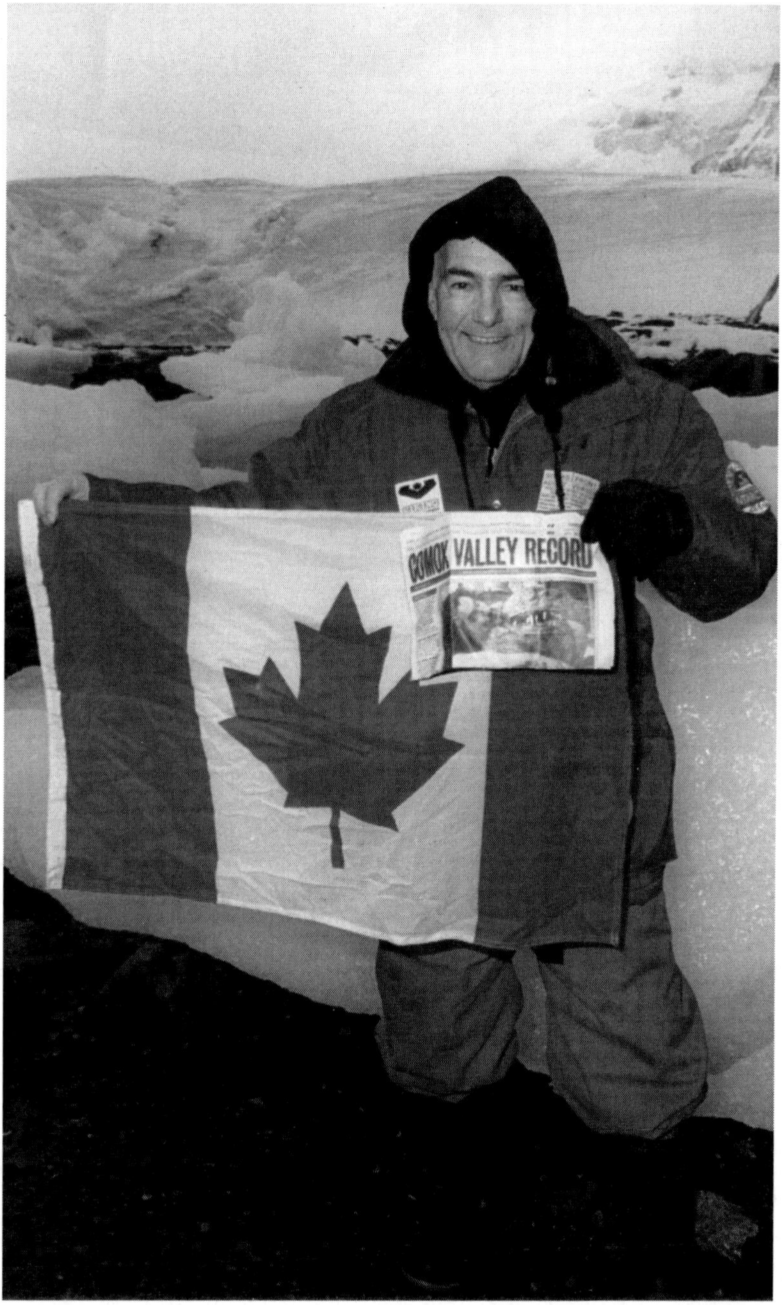
VALLEY RECORD

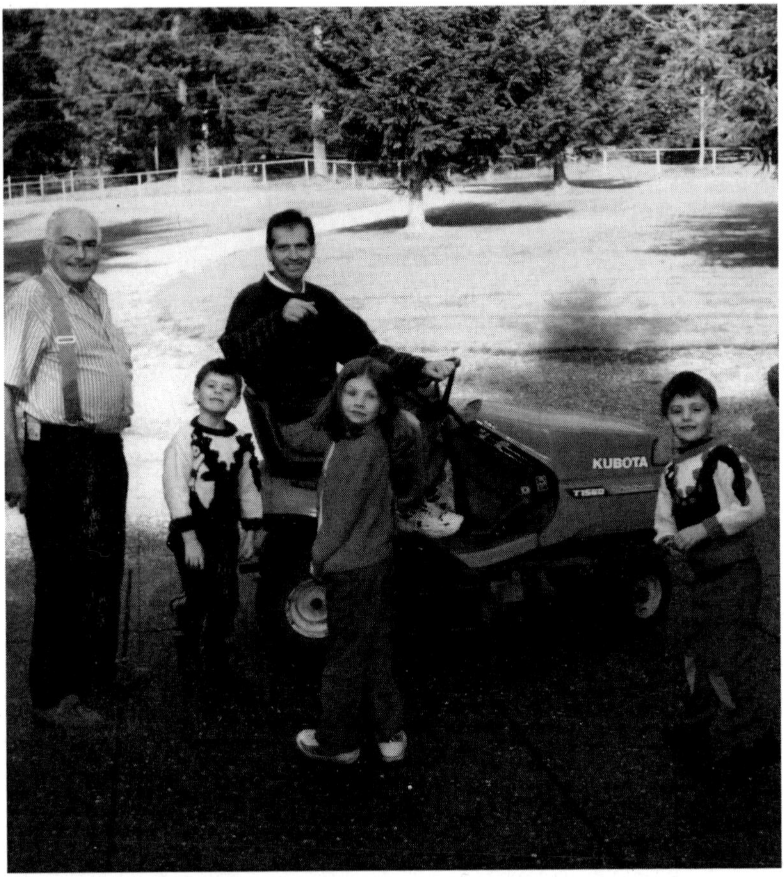

Dave with his Aussie grandchildren (L-R) Nick, Vanessa and Matt, and son-in-law, Michael, September 2005.

CHAPTER EIGHT

Turning Point

MONDAY, NOVEMBER 27–
THURSDAY, DECEMBER 1

The leisurely ambience of a Sunday morning pervades the Lodge. The place is basically deserted. Most patients, except those whose homes are too far away, have gone for the weekend, and many others completed their treatment plans by Friday. Over breakfast in the quiet cafeteria, Dave and Pat chat about the oddity that cancer can be dealt with on a Monday to Friday basis.

"Too bad I couldn't get our plants to grow only from Monday to Friday," Dave comments wryly. "Then we could have had our weekends off too."

Still, he is appreciating this break from trips to the lab to give blood.

Unfortunately, Dave's breakfast triggers a return of diarrhea. After the third bout he takes Imodium, complying with the detailed directives in the consent form, but he is not looking forward to the resulting constipation. With fewer people about, Dave takes his walker and gives his new shoes a workout. But this burst of physical ambition is quashed by sudden waves of dizziness and intense pain in his back. So he resigns himself to his familiar routine: nap, lunch, computer, nap, Tim Hortons, nap, supper, TV and, of course, taking all his meds plus Imodium every two hours.

Thankfully, the Imodium works immediately, and after

12 hours without diarrhea, he stops the annoyingly intrusive every-two-hours medication regimen.

* * * * *

Monday morning, Day 8, they make another trip after breakfast to the agency for a blood test, Dave pushing the walker up the little hill. Dave gets poked and siphoned and then they're back to their rented nest. The lab doesn't take much blood but the whole exercise wipes him out, dictating hours of rest for him to recover. But he is becoming a professional at that.

Before the trial began, Michele had advised Pat to keep a keen eye on Dave's blood reports. She had said that, with chemotherapy, the white blood cell count can drop significantly, which might leave Dave open to infection. After a few days of phoning Nurse Betsy for those numbers, Pat was told she could get the results herself from the desk on the sixth floor of the agency. Pat makes the additional trip to the agency part of her trek to Tim Hortons each afternoon. Today, the numbers hold steady.

Later that afternoon, while watching TV, Dave suddenly burbles up a small amount of grainy brown bits. He wipes it up with a tissue and wonders if it's the chocolate icing off the donut he ate earlier. They decide, regretfully, to forego their regular afternoon Tim Hortons treats. They'll make do with the coffee and cookies provided by the Lodge in the afternoon. It's not worth adding a stressed-out stomach to everything else.

* * * * *

At 2:30 in the morning, Pat is awakened by the sound of Dave retching. By the glow of a night light, he grabs the ice cream pail off the floor by his bed that they've been using as a used tissue bin. Amazingly, he catches every drop of the projectile vomit — a quarter of a bucket of chocolate brown sludge. Pat scrambles out of bed, hurries around to support his back and hold his forehead. The heaving subsides.

She gets a damp cloth from the bathroom to freshen his face. A fastidious man, Dave is so relieved that he has not fouled up the bed. But the return to calm is short-lived. He hobbles to the toilet and then has to go again 15 minutes later. He gets settled back in bed but begins heaving, and this time it's a clear slime. When it subsides, they decide to get him started on Imodium again.

He is able to sleep for a few hours, until Pat has to wake him for the next dose of Imodium. Fifteen minutes later, he is struck with cramping and goes to the bathroom again. When he returns to bed, he dozes off but Pat has to wake him again at 7 a.m. for more Imodium. Just sitting up causes him to vomit more clear stuff, but he is able to swallow the pill.

The same thing happens when he takes the Imodium at 9 a.m. When he's done in the bathroom, he takes his usual morning meds and they head up to the cafeteria. Dave can only manage a few bites of toast and just sips at his tea. On the way down in the elevator, a woman is clinging to the elevator wall, overcome by dizziness. Dave immediately hands her his walker and insists that she use it to get back to her room. Dave stays propped up against the wall by the elevator until Pat comes back with the walker. Before they walk away, the woman thanks Dave profusely and raves about his kindness. Pat can only agree.

That afternoon, Dave takes more Imodium and has more vomiting and diarrhea. Pat calls Nurse Betsy and tells her Dave isn't doing well. Pat is told to bring Dave over to the lab for blood work, and then to the second floor where Dr. Xavier will see him. They are glad the researchers are responding, but Pat isn't sure how she'll get Dave over there. He is so worn out and can't walk far, especially in the cold weather. The Lodge's nurse manager offers to drive them over to the agency herself, as she is just heading home.

With Dave bundled up and sitting on the little fold-out seat of his walker, Pat pushes him to the underground parking lot. Once at the agency, Pat wheels him along on the walker to the lab. They get settled among the hard vinyl seats and the fake flowers. Pat has the ice-cream bucket in her backpack, which Dave uses several times to deal with his heaving while they wait for a lab tech. Then, suddenly, he is struck with abdominal cramps. Pat shifts him into the bathroom and stays with him to make sure he is okay. Finally his name is called and the blood taken.

With Dave still on the walker seat, Pat gets him down to second floor where Nurse Betsy meets them and directs them to a packed waiting room. The only spot for Dave and the walker is under a wall-mounted fire extinguisher. Dave is bent over in agony.

"Nurse," Pat pleads, "Dave really needs to lie down. Haven't you got a bed that he can use?"

"Well, not really," she replies, "but I can put him in a treatment room." And she leads them through a rabbit warren of dingy yellow cubicles.

In the room, Pat helps Dave off the walker and up onto the hard, vinyl examining table.

The nurse takes his blood pressure and his temperature, adding, as she leaves, that Dr. Xavier will be in as soon as possible. Dave immediately lies down and curls up in the fetal position. He is shivering, his teeth chattering. Pat uses his coat as a blanket and piles on her own heavy wool coat and her scarf as well. Pat is scared. Dave is so ill, worse than after his eight hour, five-artery bypass surgery.

It seems ages before Dr. Xavier sweeps into the room with Nurse Betsy trailing behind. Without any preamble he asks Dave to sit up, but as he does Dave begins retching, spitting out a clear, sticky substance into the kidney bowl that Pat has grabbed off a side shelf and held under his chin. Dave sinks back down onto the table and gasps that he can't get up or he'll vomit.

Pat tells the doctor that Dave is taking Imodium but is still having diarrhea. Dr. Xavier says he will arrange for Dave to receive some IV hydration to counter Dave's fluid loss along with some Maxeran to deal with the vomiting. As the doctor heads to the door, Pat thanks him and blurts out, "At least something good has come of the trial."

The doctor lifts a quizzical eyebrow, asking, "Why do you say that, Mrs. Maddocks?"

She hurries on, "Well, on Saturday morning, Dave's edema — in his feet, ankles and legs — completely disappeared. We don't have to deal with elasticized stockings and he can wear real shoes again."

"That's great," the doctor says absentmindedly and then is gone. Pat is glad she remembered to tell the doctor because he hasn't actually given Dave a hands-on physical exam.

Nurse Betsy directs Pat to the sixth floor where Dave will get the IV hydration. There, they are handed off to Connie, a nurse in her 50s who projects a friendly, almost maternal competence. She helps Dave get comfortable in one of the three beige recliner chairs. For the last hour or so, they have been buried in the bowels of the agency. The large windows in this room are a welcome respite and reveal a darkening winter sky illuminated by the city lights.

Dave is drooping.

He's had a lot of intravenous sessions in the past couple of months, and it has been getting increasingly difficult to get the sessions started. His veins have rebelled. Pat mentions this to Nurse Connie, adding that a warm, moist cloth usually helps. After fetching the warm towel and a couple of warmed blankets for Dave, the nurse gets the IV started without a hitch.

Sometime during the three-hour procedure, a young nurse with bouncy energy and an Australian accent comes in and introduces herself as Diane. She is taking over for Nurse Connie. Dave and Pat recognize the Aussie twang immediately and Dave starts chatting with her about Australia and how both of their girls married Australians.

The mini-hydration session is going smoothly. Dave is starting to feel a little better, but he tells Pat there is no way that he can handle going back to the Lodge sitting on the walker. He asks her to go back to the Lodge and borrow one of the loaner wheelchairs kept in the entrance foyer. Nurse Diane promises to keep good watch over Dave.

Pat takes the walker back to their room, grabs her knitting as well as a small afghan off her bed, and gets permission to borrow a wheelchair, with footrests, as Dave had specified.

Back in the hydration room, about 6 p.m., Dave is resting his eyes and Pat is listlessly winding a ball of wool when Dr. Xavier shows up. Leaning against the door frame, he observes, "Well, the hydration seems to be helping."

"Yes, he certainly needed something to settle his system down," Pat replies.

"Are you feeling better, Dave?" Dr. Xavier asks.

Dave blinks awake, nods an acknowledgement and smiles. He doesn't have his hearing aids in, as the retching and heaving make them a nuisance.

Dr. Xavier smiles back and says, "That's good." He straightens up, turns on his heel and is gone.

"Well, that was short and sweet," Pat comments.

"I guess he's on his way home," muses Dave. "Hey, they got us in for hydration right away. It was good of him to drop by."

"You're right," she says. "That waiting room *was* packed to the gunnels."

Looking at her watch and then at the IV bag, she thinks maybe she'll get back to the Lodge in time for dinner.

It's going on seven o'clock by the time Dave is unhooked from the IV unit and tucked into the wheelchair. They navigate down the sidewalk and through the front doors of the Lodge.

Dave just wants to relax in the recliner, so Pat runs up to the cafeteria to grab some food before the kitchen closes. Along with a tray of her own food, she selects a small bowl of soup, crackers and a dish of lime Jell-O, Dave's favourite. She takes it all back to their room, but Dave won't take a bite of any of it. She reasons and wheedles, but he is adamant that his stomach can't handle food and he doesn't want to trigger the heaving that he's been dealing with for most of the day. But he agrees to drink some water and, later, some ginger ale.

That night, sitting on the walker seat at the bathroom sink, he deals with his evening meds, adding the new one, Dr. Xavier's prescription for Maxeran tablets, to the lineup and completing his night routine. Pat notices Dave's legs and feet are really cold. In bed, she massages his feet, first warming the creamy lotion in her hands. She has brought along an electric heating pad, which she sets on low, wraps in a towel and puts at the bottom of his bed to warm it up. She kneels on the floor beside the bed. Dave's propped up on two pillows. She snakes an arm under his pillow, leans in and hugs him.

He gently takes her face in his hands, looks in her eyes and says, "It's been a hell of a day, Bridget. Thank you."

She hugs him again and whispers, "Absolutely no problem, Sid."

Pat stands up and walks over to the oxygen condenser, clicks it on, stretches out the tubing and hands him the nasal cannula, which he positions in his nostrils, closing his eyes. Turning out his reading light she says, "Goodnight, sweetie." But he is already asleep.

She pulls the privacy drape, just a little, to create shade for the reading light over her bed. Changing her mind about trying to read, she sits in the dark, her back against the headboard, hugging her knees to her chest.

It's still early, but she makes the sign of the Cross and begins silently mouthing the few prayers she says most nights. She starts with "Our Father," which for years has been her plea to God to look after Dave. She has always reserved this most powerful of supplications for her husband. Tonight, she prays it slowly, fervently.

Hot tears leak out of the corner of her eyes. She brushes them away with the flat of her hands. This is not the time to lose it. The researchers have responded. They are aware of Dave's difficulties and Dave seems much better tonight than he has all day.

* * * * *

That night, Day 10 of the trial, Wednesday, Pat uses Dave's little travel alarm clock to make sure Dave gets the increasing number of medications on time, charting them to keep everything organized.

Groggy, Dave is not thrilled to be woken up for medicine. Almost immediately after his suppository, Nurse Connie's suggestion, his gut starts cramping. Pat is up and able to move all the oxygen paraphernalia out of the way as Dave makes a break for the toilet using the walker for support. By the time his body settles down and he is back in bed, he drinks down the Maxeran pills and easily falls asleep.

When it's time for the next dose, Pat is still awake. Again the suppository triggers diarrhea, and now Dave has a fever. Pat's been checking his temperature every day, again relieved that she remembered to pack a thermometer so they can follow the trial instructions to inform the researchers if his temperature goes above 39 degrees Celsius.

Dave manages to do his morning ablutions, supported by the walker, and takes his regular morning meds, but then his gut goes into spasm. Pat insists on taking his temperature again. It is now higher than 39. Immediately, Pat calls Nurse Betsy. She asks about Dave's vomiting and Pat tells her that, so far, there has been nothing since yesterday afternoon's visit with Dr. Xavier but she also says that the Imodium hasn't stopped his diarrhea. Pat suggests that the suppositories recommended by the Daycare nurse might be triggering these episodes. Pat also mentions that Dave hasn't eaten anything since yesterday morning. Nurse Betsy says she'll report to Dr. Xavier and get back to them.

She does – within just a few minutes. She tells Pat to stop the suppositories but to keep on with the Maxeran. She says that Dr. Xavier has ordered Cipro, that she has phoned the prescription into the drugstore down on Broadway and they have it ready for Pat to pick up now.

That bit of news takes Pat by surprise. Cipro is a very ordinary antibiotic, not at all as potent as Ketek, the one that

Dave had lately been stepped up to. Pat says as much to Nurse Betsy. The trial nurse merely says that Cipro is the one that the doctor ordered. If an antibiotic has been prescribed, that must mean Dave has a bacterial infection, but if the remedy is so ordinary, Pat reasons, the infection must be something he can easily fight off. Her concerns fade.

Nurse Betsy asks if Dave is drinking lots of fluids and Pat assures her that he is, pointing out that with all the medication he has to take, plus the Imodium every two hours, he drinks lots of water.

"Is he getting at least eight ounces *an hour*?" the nurse persists.

Pat is taken aback.

"Well, no, not *that* much. That's like a coffee mug full every hour!"

"Yes," says Nurse Betsy, "that's what he needs to take in. So go and pick up that prescription, get Dave started on it and see how he does today."

Pat gets off the phone and tells Dave about the antibiotics and the amount of liquid he must consume. Dave groans.

"Damn," Dave exclaims. "I must have some sort of bug. I thought we'd done a good job of avoiding contact with people."

"I think we did, Dave," Pat commiserates. "Hey, bacteria are everywhere. Really, there was no way to eliminate them from our lives. It's not our fault, Sid. Let's get you started on the Cipro. If you drink a full glass of something every time you take one of your medications, you should nail that eight ounces thing."

But when she places the first antibiotic pill in his hand, Dave is incensed.

"Goddamned horse pill!" he complains. "I told them I could manage swallowing everything except big pills!" He pops it in his mouth and drinks it down but it is a painful exercise for his cancer-ridden esophagus.

Pat offers him a yogurt cup, but he pushes it away. "You know I don't like that stuff."

"But it's a good idea to take it when you're on an antibiotic," she counters.

"Look," he snaps. "You know I hate yogurt and there's no way my stomach can handle it. Forget it!"

A sullen silence follows. Then Dave is seized with cramps. He hauls himself out of the soft chair and wheels his walker into the bathroom. It is a long session. He asks Pat to bring two pillows and to position the walker, with its seat down in front of him on the toilet so he can lean on it, rest his head for the duration.

From home, Pat has brought a couple of pairs of slippers — terry-towel hotel ones emblazoned with "The Ritz Carlton." She's had them warming on the radiator and now slips a pair on his feet. The tile floor is achingly cold. She covers his back with his viyella robe.

He heads for bed to recover. But just minutes later, apologetically, Pat reminds him it's time for another Imodium. He takes the pills, but only one swig of ginger ale.

Lunch is being served in the cafeteria but Dave refuses to consider eating. He's comfortable and wants to sleep so Pat goes up for a bite alone. She knows he needs a break from her constant presence.

As Pat is coming out of the elevator, returning from lunch, she sees Michele signing in at the reception desk. They embrace and Pat says how surprised she is to see Michele out and about. She's had pneumonia and has been unable to visit.

"Well, I'm not quite better yet," she says. "I'll just poke my head in the room and say hi to Dad."

She briefly greets her dad, then Pat and Michele walk to the lounge. Michele asks how Dave is doing and Pat tells her that he was vomiting a lot yesterday but that he got three hours of IV, that he's on Maxeran now and that Cipro was added this morning.

Michele cuts her off saying, "It sounds like they've got a good handle on things." The conversation turns to what's new with her boys and all her difficulties setting up house. Dave is sleeping when Pat returns to the room. She wakes him and hands him the next dose, telling him that he must drink a whole glass of *something*, as she can see that he hasn't touched any of the ginger ale she'd left for him while she was at lunch.

He is just sinking back to sleep when he suddenly blinks awake and asks her to quickly help him into the bathroom. He just needs her arm for support and he makes it to the toilet in time. Another long session with walker, pillows, robe, warm slippers. But, happily, his temperature is down.

Before he falls asleep, Pat gets him to drink some water and then tucks the afghan around him and kisses his forehead. She goes out for some groceries, hoping she can tempt him with Chicken-In-A-Mug or his favourite Ritz crackers. When she gets back, Dave is fast asleep. She knows he's not getting enough liquid, so she starts disturbing him every 15 minutes to get him to drink. He goes along with this plan and takes the Imodium and Maxeran along with it. She persuades him to sit in the recliner. He is unable to focus on the TV or his computer. He just wants to doze.

But later that night, he is in the bathroom with diarrhea again. It's bad this time. Still, every two hours, Pat is rousing him to take medicine. And every 15 minutes, she's bothering him to drink so she can get enough fluids into him. For Dave, Pat's constant shoulder-shaking is highly annoying, and they are both dispirited.

Cajoling him onto the seat of his walker, Pat wheels him into the bathroom. She convinces him to tell her exactly what meds he uses, morning and night. She writes it out in the order that he likes so that she can lay it all out for him. It's another ego-bruising handover of a task that is truly his; Dave has usually set out her sleeping pill for her each night, as well as his own meds. Earlier, she had bought a paring knife and then had quartered the large Cipro pill, nipping off the little sharp corners; he's noticed this nicety and thanked her.

When he's back in bed, she massages his feet and gets him to sip some ginger ale before he falls fast asleep.

Pat leaves Dave sleeping and goes down to the activity room to email an update to their daughter Lisa. She hates having to type up her personal thoughts in the middle of a room full of strangers but it only takes a few minutes to type up a summary of her worries.

She makes herself a cup of tea, grabs a sandwich and starts back to their room. She notices an elderly couple coming into the Lodge, wrestling with the heavy outer door. She knows the old man is receiving radiation. Pat shakes her head wondering how, at their age, they can handle all the daily, soul-destroying catastrophes that seem inherent to fighting cancer. She knows that her ability to cope is fast crumbling.

The nurse on duty comes up to Pat and hugs her shoulder. She asks how Dave is doing.

"Not good at all," Pat replies.

The nurse gives Pat's shoulder another squeeze and says, "Well, you make sure you take care of yourself." And she heads back to her office.

"She's totally tuned out!" Pat mutters to herself. She wasn't the one that needed a hug.

Back in their dimly lit room, she updates her makeshift record sheet and figures out when Dave must take the next dose of pills. She sets the alarm clock for 3 a.m. They are going to have to try harder tomorrow.

* * * * *

Dave's reliable little travel clock wakes Pat. It's Day 11 of the trial, December 1. She gently shakes Dave awake and hands him his pills. He drinks almost a whole glass of water downing the four pills. He has no problem going back to sleep.

Not so for Pat. She is expecting Dave's body to react, to either retch or cramp, and her every nerve is tensed, ready to assist. But Dave sleeps on. At 4:30 a.m., just as her brain is mellowing, Dave calls out to her, urgently asking for help to the bathroom. He leans against her as he shuffles across the carpet and onto the cold tiles and then eases himself onto the toilet. Pat sets up the walker for him to rest on and puts the warmed slippers on his cold feet.

Dave uses the walker to come back to bed, gets halfway there and returns to the toilet.

Pat does everything again to keep him warm. A half hour later, his body has ceased cramping and he can get back into bed. Instantly, he is asleep.

Four hours later, Pat is still wide awake. It's time, again, for pills. Dave takes them and falls back to sleep. But an hour later, his gut cramping, he rushes to the toilet. This time, Dave needs Pat to fully support him when he walks. A firm arm to cling to is no longer enough.

Before 9 a.m., Pat calls Nurse Betsy.

"We gave it a day," Pat says, "and Dave is no better. This morning, he has already had three bouts of diarrhea. Yesterday, he had seven. His temperature is down but only to 101.5 F. He hasn't been vomiting but this is the third day that he hasn't eaten any food — he's got nothing to bring up and nothing to form a bowel movement; it's just liquid. He is drinking but it is difficult to get eight ounces an hour into him as he wants to sleep so much."

Because the vomiting seems to be under control, Nurse Betsy suggests Dave reduce the Maxeran to one pill every six hours and she tells Pat to bring Dave to the lab at 2:15 that afternoon for more blood work and hydration. When Pat relays the plan to Dave, he wearily nods his head in acceptance.

She tries, again, to sell him on the idea of something light to eat from the breakfast bar, but he just tells her to go get something for herself — not to bring anything back for him.

Before she leaves, she puts a juice box with a straw on his night stand and asks him to drink it while she is gone. He is sound asleep when she gets back 15 minutes later, but the juice box is empty. She's grateful and relieved. But it's temporary.

Soon after his next round of medication, he needs her help to the toilet — again. They are both increasingly frustrated and exhausted. But when this attack is finished, he lets Pat wash him at the sink and he runs the electric razor over his grey stubble.

He says he doesn't want to get dressed until they need to go out, that he wants to stay in bed. So she bargains with him. If he doesn't take the drink she offers him every hour, she'll keep offering it to him, bit by bit, until it's empty.

"The more you can drink at one time the less often I'll have to disturb you. What do you want to drink this hour?"

"Just water," he grinds out.

She measures out a mug of water. He drinks half and snuggles down into the bed.

Before the appointment, she gets Dave up to get dressed. He's very weak, but he can still dress himself. He just needs help with his socks and shoes. They hurry to the agency, Pat wheeling him through the winter winds. Blood samples taken, they go up to the sixth floor and are taken into the hydration room right away. There is another patient receiving treatment and they make small talk with him, but he is soon finished and Pat and Dave are alone. A nurse pops in occasionally, but it is up to Pat to transfer him and the IV pole to the bathroom.

After a while, Pat checks with the reception desk to see if today's blood report is available. She is told to see Nurse Betsy. She takes the elevator and finds her tucked away down the hall on the fourth floor. She willingly prints off the blood report for Pat.

"Dave is really, really sick," Pat tells Nurse Betsy. "He's still not eating and he's sleeping a lot with seven to ten bouts of diarrhea a day. Today is Thursday, and Dave is scheduled for more CPX-1 on Tuesday. I just don't see how he is going to be well enough to take the next dose. But we'll give it until tomorrow to see if what's being done today will make a difference. If it doesn't, he'll have to cancel the Tuesday session."

Nurse Betsy says she understands and will tell Dr. Xavier.

Pat gets back to the hydration room in time to give Dave his next Imodium pill. Another bout of diarrhea to deal with; wrestling with the IV pole merely adds more angst. Dave is exhausted from all the maneuvering. Back at the Lodge, Pat restarts the parade of fluid and medication offerings.

The 10 p.m. dose triggers another bout of diarrhea. This time, Dave is too wrung out to attempt his evening medication routine, so Pat brings it all to his night table, handing him each pill, turbo inhaler, tablet and puffer in the right sequence. She finagles him into allowing her to give him a sponge bath and she hopes the warm soapy water will give him some comfort.

The late evening double dose of Imodium is followed at midnight by yet another session on the toilet. Once Dave is again tucked into bed, his oxygen cannula hissing quietly, Pat is able to grab a snack from the activity room and get herself ready for bed. Setting the alarm for 3 a.m., she falls into a fitful sleep.

CHAPTER NINE
Trauma
FRIDAY, DECEMBER 2, AND SATURDAY, DECEMBER 3

At 2:00 a.m., Pat wakes up in the dark to the sound of shuffling. Dave's hand is scrabbling over the nightstand. He is looking for something.

"What are you doing?" Pat asks.

"I'm looking for a drink," he says.

"Great," she says.

Pat is thrilled. His hand wraps around a juice box that she had left there for him. He sucks on the little straw eagerly, drains the container and slides back down in his bed, falling asleep instantly.

Glancing at the clock, she realizes she has only half an hour before she has to wake him up again for his Imodium. She lies awake in the blackness, quietly rejoicing that he has, finally, *wanted* to drink something. Now if only he would eat something. Suddenly she thinks of Boost, berating herself for forgetting about the fortified drink packed with nutrition. She switches into action mode, wondering if the Lodge might have some. She gets up, pulls on her robe and walks down the hall to the office.

The night nurse tells her they do have something similar and offers Pat a six-pack of Carnation Breakfast that she has in the little fridge in her office. Pat takes them back to their room and when she wakes Dave for his medication, she encourages him to try the liquid food. He drinks half the container and falls asleep. When she wakes him again four hours later, he finishes the container while taking the next dose of Imodium. But Pat's elation is flattened when he tells her the stuff is too sweet, that it makes him nauseous. Even worse, his gut goes into spasms and he is forced to deal with more diarrhea which strikes hard, twice in half an hour.

At 9:00 a.m., Pat phones Nurse Betsy to tell her about Dave's condition. She gets the usual directive — blood test and hydration; same time, same place, that afternoon. Pat conveys the message to Dave. Those remedies have so far proven useless, and to repeat the exhausting process doesn't feel like much of a plan. Dave consents, but he is weary.

Pat asks Dave if he wants help getting out of bed to do his morning meds or if he'd prefer she bring everything over to him in bed.

"Forget it, Pat," he says, with a sigh. "I can't face it now. Maybe later."

She is ready to launch into a passionate objection when the telephone rings. It's Nurse Betsy. She says Dr. Xavier wants Dave to provide a stool sample and bring it to the lab — right away. Nurse Betsy tells Pat she can pick up the container at the agency lab. When Pat hangs up and tells Dave, he looks rueful. His voice is tired when he replies, "Well, could you help me to the bathroom first? My blasted gut is churning."

She quickly reaches her arm around his back and helps him hobble into the bathroom. She's basically carrying him. His legs have no strength.

"Oh, babe," she says. "I'm so sorry. Not again!"

"Don't worry," he wheezes. "I'm sure it will happen again so the doctor can get his sample."

After his bowels finally calm down, Pat gets Dave settled back in bed and administers his Imodium — it's due again. He drinks well and falls asleep. Pat puts on her coat and walks quickly over to the lab. A bulky bundle is waiting for her at the lab's reception desk. She is mystified. Why would Dr. Xavier wait days to request a sample when he's already prescribed an antibiotic? But what does she know? He's the expert.

Dave's prediction comes true. Shortly after she returns to their room, he's hit with another attack of diarrhea. She collects his sample and gets him back to bed. He falls asleep quickly and she throws on her coat and hurries the sample over to the lab. She is back in time to disturb Dave for more fluid and Imodium. Another session of painful cramps and sitting on the toilet ensues.

In the afternoon, getting ready to go to the agency, she has to help Dave get dressed. For the first time, he's too weak to do any of it himself. She notices his body has changed. It seems saggy and, when he sits in the wheelchair, he looks so frail, crumpled and very white.

It is going on 2:30 p.m. when the lab tech finishes draining his blood into a small vial; Pat wheels Dave to the sixth floor for more hydration. The waiting room is a sea of ailing humanity. The wheelchair is much too large to fit in there, so Pat positions it at the entrance, immediately adjacent to the door to the hydration room. Strangely, the hydration room is empty. After waiting for about an hour, with Dave slumped over in his wheelchair, half asleep, Pat has to go to the bathroom. She decides to use the one in the empty hydration room right behind them, so she'll only be away from Dave for a minute. But as she walks in, a petite young nurse Pat hasn't met bustles up. "The room is contaminated. You're not allowed in here," she scolds. "If you need a bathroom, use the one around the corner and down the hall on the right."

The nurse closes the heavy fire door firmly behind her. Pat quickly finds the other bathroom and she's back beside Dave in less than two minutes. He is still sleeping.

The nurse is having a bad day. Pat hears her arguing heatedly on the phone at the reception desk. Then Pat sees Nurse Diane, Dave's nurse from last Tuesday, urging the agitated little nurse to go home and offering to take over, to get Dave's IV started. Then the young Aussie nurse comes over and asks them to come into the now open hydration room.

Pat comments that the other nurse said it was contaminated. Nurse Diane laughs, "Oh, she blew it all out of proportion. A cleaning crew has fixed the problem."

Pat and Nurse Diane help Dave out of the wheelchair and into the recliner. Pat parks the monster wheelchair just outside the door. Again, Pat suggests a warm cloth to help get the IV port established. When Nurse Diane leaves to get a towel, Pat points out to Dave that it's already almost 4:00 p.m. It's Friday and they know that the agency "goes dark" on the weekend. No one has told them what the plan is for Dave's care over the weekend. Pat worries that the trial nurse might be going home soon, so she wants to go down to speak to her. Dave nods his head in agreement. As soon as Nurse Diane comes back, Pat heads for the elevators.

Walking down the hallway on the fourth floor, Pat passes Dr. Xavier, lounging against the wall, talking with a woman in a white lab coat who is sporting glitzy glasses. Pat nods her head towards him as she passes, but Dr. Xavier is involved in his conversation.

Pat finds Nurse Betsy in her cubicle and asks her if today's results from Dave's blood tests are in. She taps on her computer; his results aren't there. Pat suddenly bursts into tears.

"Dave is so sick, so weak," she says between sobs. "There's no way he can continue with the trial. No way he's having the next infusion on Tuesday. He's starting to hate me and push me away because I'm always in his face. And I have to be. I'm constantly begging him to drink."

She is wracked with sorrow because she knows Dave will be so disappointed in himself for not being able to carry on with the trial. She knows how much Dave wanted to help.

Pat asks Nurse Betsy if they have a care plan for Dave to cover Saturday and Sunday. The trial nurse says she will ask

Dr. Xavier and goes out to the hall. When she comes back, she says Dr. Xavier is briefing the doctor who is taking over for him for the next two days, and that she'll go back in a few minutes to find out what the plan is for Dave. Nurse Betsy gets back on the computer, finds the blood report and prints it off. The two women are just looking at one another.

"This is stupid," says Pat, impatiently. "I'm going out there to talk to him."

Pat marches up to the two doctors, apologizes for interrupting and says, speaking slowly and firmly, "Dr. Xavier, the Imodium just isn't working. Dave —"

Before she can say anything more, Dr. Xavier says forcefully, "Well, then, take him off it."

Pat feels like she's been punched in the gut, the wind knocked out of her. "Are you sure?" she manages to ask. "I've been working so hard all week to get it into him."

"Take him off it," Dr. Xavier repeats imperiously.

Pat stands there in stunned silence while Dr. Xavier introduces a tall, heavily built man beside him as Dr. Zachary, the resident oncologist who will be covering for Dr. Xavier over the weekend. Dr. Xavier then turns to Dr. Zachary and assures him that he will be available on his cell. He continues talking to Dr. Zachary saying something about bringing Dave back to the agency tomorrow for another blood test and more hydration. They ignore Pat. She mumbles "Thanks" before heading back to the bank of elevators.

When Pat walks back into the hydration room, Dave looks terrible, almost beat up. There is an older nurse tweaking the tape holding the IV needle in the back of Dave's hand. Pat looks askance at the nurse.

The nurse says, "I've got the saline drip started now. The other girls tried three times but couldn't get the vein. They called me. I'm an IV specialist."

"It isn't a great IV port," she adds. "I've had to use a butterfly."

Pat tells the nurse that Dave will probably be coming back tomorrow for another hydration session.

"That's good to know," she replies. "I'll make sure the staff here knows about that, to save the site."

As she leaves, Pat sincerely thanks the woman and Dave manages to nod his head, smiling wanly. Pat tells Dave that Dr. Xavier told her to stop giving the Imodium. But she can see he is tired from the marathon poking session he's just been through, and she urges him to sleep.

Later, Nurse Diane returns and tells them they are to come back tomorrow morning to the lab and then to a different area of the sixth floor for hydration. The unit they're in now will be closed over the weekend. Suddenly, the agency seems eerily quiet. It's hard to believe it is the same place that was so crowded just two hours earlier.

Through the window, Pat and Dave watch the snowflakes drift down. Pat worries about getting back to the Lodge. It is already dark and there is a light skiff of snow on the ground.

About 5:30 p.m., Nurse Diane informs them they are closing in an hour, but Dave's IV won't be done. She suggests they either cut the session short, as they are coming back for more in the morning, or she can draw up the transfer papers and move them to 6 West, another area on the same floor, to finish off the bag.

Pat looks at Dave. She asks wryly, "We're not doing anything tonight, are we, Dave?"

His gaunt but handsome face breaks into a smile.

"Dave needs all the fluid he can get," says Pat. "We'll move to 6 West."

Pat helps Nurse Diane shift Dave from the hydration recliner into the big wheelchair. With his IV pouch swinging on its hook, a lifeline of plastic tubing tethered to his arm, Pat rolls Dave through the deserted hallways. Nurse Diane, guiding the IV machine, shows them the way. The sign on the doorway demands strict adherence to thorough handwashing in the bank of metal troughs in the ante-room. They wash their hands and then wrestle with the next set of heavy fire doors. Nurse Diane turns Dave and his transfer papers over to a nurse at the reception desk and leaves. The new ward seems disorganized — the hallways are lined with carts, piled high with linens and stacks of vinyl chairs. The nurse explains the area is being renovated and she escorts them to a small room at the end of a hall that is packed with furniture. But there's a TV, a well-stocked snack area and a bathroom. The nurse sets Dave up in a recliner.

Pat tries again to interest Dave in eating, even just a cracker. He refuses, but he does take a few sips of 7-Up. Pat grabs a sandwich. Just after 7:30 p.m., the IV is finished. The nurse detaches the tubing and bandages the port site. But as Dave moves from the recliner to the wheelchair, his body goes into spasm. Pat supports him into the little cubbyhole of a bathroom. There's not much to be grateful for, just lately, but not having the IV pole to contend with is a relief. Dave isn't losing a lot of fluid, but each gut-wrenching incident is an enormous drain on his stamina.

Exiting 6 West, Pat manages to get Dave and the bulky wheelchair through the heavy double doors. They encounter no one as they make their way through the agency, out the front doors and into the bitterly cold night. The fat rubber tires of the monster wheelchair make it easy to steer on the snowy sidewalks.

Back in their room, Pat helps Dave towards the bed, but with all the jostling, his bowels begin churning. He is forced to remain on the toilet for the next hour and a half. Pat gets the walker and pillows in place, the warmed slippers on his feet and drapes his robe around his hunched body. Almost exactly every 15 minutes, he is hit with pain. Pat tries to get Dave to take some of his meds, but he is in agony and won't even consider it.

He was probably right to refuse, for his stomach continues to roil. Pat hands him the bathroom's metal trash basket. He vomits.

Eventually, his body quiets down. Pat disassembles the makeshift cocoon to get Dave onto the walker. It is obvious to both of them that Dr. Xavier's order to quit the Imodium was wrong. While the drug hadn't halted the diarrhea, it had made it less frequent. Dave agrees to restart the Imodium, to take the initial dose of two pills, but he is adamant that he will take *nothing* else — none of his regular meds.

"I just want to sleep!" he pleads.

Though she wants to argue, she can't refuse him. Pat undresses him, folds him into his bed with the electric heating pad for his cold feet, positions the hissing oxygen cannula in his nose, gives him a hug and kisses his forehead. He is aware of none of these ministrations. Sleep has overtaken him.

In the gloom, Pat sits on the edge of her bed, perplexed and deeply disturbed. She is scared for Dave now. Nobody seems to understand or acknowledge how ill he is. She begins to suspect that perhaps Dr. Xavier doesn't know much about CPX-1 and managing the infection that Dave is contending with. Then she begins to doubt herself. Both Nurse Betsy and Dr. Xavier seem unconcerned with Dave's condition. And yet, how can Dave be expected to endure such agony with so little help? She wonders why — despite her many reports to the trial nurse that Dave was experiencing diarrhea 10 times a day, basically every time he moved, that he was too weak to move, that he hadn't eaten since Tuesday — no one seems to think any of this is significant.

At 10:00 p.m., with Dave asleep, she grabs their cell phone, quietly slips out of the room and goes to the empty front lounge to call her sister Jackie, a retired nurse. She isn't home. Pat doesn't leave a message, not wanting a return phone call to disturb Dave. And she is unsure just how to phrase her concerns. Pat stands there, wracking her brains, trying to think who else she can talk to about her fears for Dave. She knows Michele is in bed by 9:30 p.m. and her friend Nurse Alexis and her husband are away on vacation. Contacting the after-hours number of the agency would be a huge risk. She is worried that calling them would be taken as criticism and that Dave might get *less* attention.

The Lodge's night nurse, walking back to her office, notices Pat and comes over.

"You're looking worried," she comments.

Pat is overwhelmed by this small gesture of interest. Tears well up and she croaks out, "Oh, God, I'm so worried! Dave is *so* sick!"

The nurse hauls Pat to her ample bosom, stokes her back and says, "Things will look better in the morning, dear. You go and get some rest." Then she continues on her way.

Yet again, Pat's self-doubt about her understanding of the state of Dave's health surfaces. Maybe she is overreacting. She and Dave don't know much about chemotherapy. Maybe what Dave is going through is normal. The thought of the suffering that cancer patients must be enduring tears at her heart. She mentally shakes herself. Maybe the night nurse is right. Dave has a new doctor in the morning. Maybe he will be more help.

She tiptoes into their room. Dave is sound asleep. She gets ready for bed and updates her record sheet of Dave's diarrhea occurrences and medications given. Dave's nightly doubled dose of Imodium is due at 11:00 and then again at 3 a.m. She sets the little alarm clock.

Dave wakes at 11, vomiting. When his system calms down, he is able to take his pills, but soon after, he must cope with another stomach upheaval. Still, somehow the medicine manages to stay down and he is able to go back to sleep. And so, too, can Pat.

Not for long. A couple of hours later, Dave is up, needing the bathroom. This time, he cannot walk at all, even with Pat's help. She needs the walker to move him, and he needs help cleaning himself off. They both sleep until 5:00 a.m., when he wakes up needing the bathroom again.

This bout over, she wipes his bum and gets him tucked back in bed, both of them now almost accustomed to the humiliation.

Dave sleeps off and on, between interruptions, until they must get ready to go over to the agency. For the third time, Dave refuses to take his regular morning and night meds. He will only take the Imodium — which triggers another bout of diarrhea just as they are going out the door.

It's Saturday, 9:15 a.m. The agency is dark, silent and empty. No one is around, not even cleaning staff. Pat and Dave make their way to the lab on the third floor. The lights are off in the deserted waiting room, but watery winter sunlight floods in through the windows. A lab tech bustles in, apologizing profusely for making them wait, then quickly takes Dave's blood.

Again, Pat is impressed by the courtesy they have received in this area of the agency and she says just that to Dave as she pushes him in the wheelchair towards the elevators. "Sid, of all the professionals that we have encountered in this building, the lab techs have always been consistently thoughtful and kind."

Arriving at 6 West, which they would never have found if they hadn't been taken there last night, they enter the ward and one of the nurses escorts them to a semi-private room that is in the process of being dismantled. Now there is just the one bed — next to the window — and an orange vinyl chair, which leaves lots of room to park the big wheelchair. The privacy drapes for the room have been removed and the ceiling railing, which has been partly unbolted, is hanging askew. The nurse helps Dave up onto the bed and connects his IV through the saved butterfly port. She tells them it will take three hours to complete the session and asks if he would like a warm blanket.

"Yes, please," he says, in a raspy voice. When she doesn't return, Pat goes out to remind her and asks if Dr. Zachary is expected to come in.

"Yes, he'll be doing rounds in an hour or so."

"Great," says Pat, relieved. "Could you ask him to drop in to talk to Dave and me? And could we have a jug of water and a couple of glasses, please?"

"Sure thing," says the nurse, handing Pat some hot flannel sheets. After tucking them around Dave, Pat sits at the foot of the bed and starts knitting. Dave is lying on the bed, dozing in the sun now streaming through the window. The saline droplets course through the plastic tubing into the back of his hand.

Pat has brought the Imodium with her. His next dose is due. The glasses and jug of water haven't arrived, but Pat finds some disposable cups in the bathroom. Within minutes of swallowing the pill, Dave's gut starts cramping and he urgently needs the toilet. The response time of the nurses has been pathetic, so they automatically deal with it themselves. He manages to swing himself to the edge of the bed, but he is so weak, there is no way he can walk that far. Somehow he puts his arm on Pat's shoulder; she grabs him around his waist and directs the IV pole, and they crabwalk over to the toilet — making it just in time.

With so much exertion, Dave is instantly asleep once he's back on the bed and covered up. Pat goes back to trying to concentrate on knitting the toque. Just before noon, Dr. Zachary comes into their room.

Pat stands up in greeting and introduces him to Dave. Dr. Zachary nods at Dave and takes Pat's place on the lone chair.

Pat immediately tells Dr. Zachary that Dave is back on Imodium. She tells him that she had stopped giving it to Dave as Dr. Xavier had ordered her to do yesterday afternoon, but that last night had been a disaster; that Dave had four liquid bowel movements in just an hour and a half and had a huge vomiting session. Since being back on Imodium, she says, Dave's diarrhea episodes are back to once every two hours or so.

Dr. Zachary makes no comment. He glances at the paper in his hand and begins to tell them about the results of the blood test from that morning. He says Dave's creatinine level has gone up to 250. Pat gasps. On the lab report she got from Nurse Betsy the day before, the creatinine had risen almost 35 percent above Dave's normal level. Now the doctor is saying that yesterday's worrying level has doubled!

Alarm bells go off in Pat's mind. She's remembering her Mom's ICU nurse saying that if the kidneys reach a creatinine level of 300, they are irreparably damaged and can shut down. At this dizzying rate of increase, Dave is in huge danger.

Directing this information to Dave, Dr. Zachary says he can't admit him to the hospital because there are no beds but that he will consult a kidney expert. Dr. Zachary then asks Dave what medications he is taking.

Dave's panicked eyes meet Pat's and mirror her concern that maybe Dr. Zachary hasn't looked at Dave's patient record. The lengthy list of Dave's daily medications, all the emergency remedies and even a short medical history are all organized on a neatly typed, single sheet of paper back at the Lodge. She never thought she needed to bring them. She knows the agency has a copy in Dave's file.

Dave's raspy voice is listing off his meds hesitantly, stumbling over the pronunciations. This frightens Pat. Dave is a genius at managing his meds; he's normally able to list them off so easily. She comes up with a couple that he's missed. But Dr. Zachary cuts her off and says to Dave, "Well, you should stop taking any medication that could injure your kidneys. The Vasotec, the antibiotic, the Aspirin."

"But Dr. Xavier just put Dave on the antibiotic, Cipro, a couple days ago. Why would he put Dave on a drug that could harm his kidneys?" Pat asks.

Dr. Zachary doesn't answer her question.

"Actually, Dr. Zachary," Pat persists, "Dave is way ahead of you. He has refused the last three doses of his daily meds."

Dr. Zachary stands up to leave. Turning to Dave, he tells him to come back the next day for more blood work and hydration. The nurse who set Dave up with the IV comes into the room shortly after Dr. Zachary leaves, replacing the almost empty saline bag with a full one. She informs them that

Dr. Zachary has added it to Dr. Xavier's order, which will take about another hour or so to finish and that they are to come back tomorrow morning, same time, same place.

The hydration session wears on. Dave drifts in and out of sleep. He no longer needs a blanket. The sun, magnified by the large window, is surprisingly hot for a winter's day. When he takes his Imodium, again it sets him off and they must repeat the perilous and clumsy trip to the bathroom. They are successful but they both have an even greater appreciation of the little walker that they have so come to rely on.

Down the hall, the nursing station sounds like a raucous hen party. Pat can hear one of them phoning around to see if someone can fill a next-day, Sunday, shift. Every time she hangs up, she tells the other women at the nursing station what excuse had been given for not taking the shift. Gales of laughter and snide comments ensue each time.

When the new bag of IV fluid is done, the nurse comes in to bandage Dave's IV port so it can be used again tomorrow. She says it's precarious and hopes it will last. Pat wheels Dave back down the hill to the Lodge, and when they get back to their room, the diarrhea won't stop. Almost every hour, he must be trundled to the toilet. Dave is barely awake, resting his head on the pillows on the walker's seat, unable to leave the bathroom for more than 15 minutes. Pat tries to offer sips of water or ginger ale. He refuses everything.

When she finally gets him back to bed, he sits on the edge, unsure about whether to go to the bathroom again. When Pat gently asks him what he wants to do — get back into bed or go to the toilet — his answer is garbled. But he doesn't complain, doesn't break down. He just sits there in a daze of confusion.

Pat is frantic. She can't think what to do to make Dave comfortable, to ease the agony of the constant cramping and heaving of his emaciated body. Nothing she does stops his suffering. She paces back and forth in the room, between the beds and the dresser, her mind searching for options that might rescue Dave from this nightmare.

In the midst of this turmoil, the phone rings. It's Michele, on her first day back at work. She's on a coffee break and is calling to see how her dad is. Pat feels a surge of relief: this is someone who will believe her. Pat tells her Dave is sitting on the bed unable to decide whether to lie down or go to the bathroom, that the hourly diarrhea episodes have made him so weak that he can no longer stand by himself, that she has to get him to the toilet on the walker, that she has to wake him up two to three times every hour and beg him to drink so she can get enough fluids into him, that he hasn't eaten for five days, that the mini hydration sessions aren't helping, that Dr. Zachary has told them to come back in the morning for another session and it is all so useless, Dave just keeps getting worse.

Michele asks if she has called Dr. Zachary to tell him about Dave's confusion. Pat admits that she hasn't.

"You've got to do that, Mom," she says. "It's important. He needs to know what's happening."

Pat tells Michele she doesn't think Dr. Zachary will listen to her; that she felt like he was dismissing everything she had told him earlier today.

"Mom," Michele insists. "Promise me you'll call him as soon as I get off the phone. You've got his number?"

Pat says she has the after-hours number for the agency and agrees to call.

Just as Michele is saying goodbye, she mentions that a commode might be helpful. Pat can't believe she hasn't thought of that before. No one at the Lodge has told her there might be one available and when she goes to find the nurse, there is no nurse on duty. The reception desk's cute young volunteer doesn't know what a commode is, but she takes Pat to a couple of closets to see if they can find one. They're packed with linens, puzzles, Christmas decorations — everything but a commode.

Pat is anxious to get back to Dave. She needs to wake him up, again. He drinks down the pill and the cramping starts.

She gets him settled on the toilet and back to bed. He drinks some water and is back to sleep. Pat picks up the phone and punches in the agency's after-hours number.

She is surprised when she's connected to a nurse in 6 West. Pat asks to speak to Dr. Zachary.

"Why?" snaps the nurse, in a brusque and off-putting voice. Pat didn't think she would have to justify her request. Being put through to 6 West worries her, as they will have Dave's name down for hydration in the morning. The nurse's attitude frightens her. Maybe she'll be judged as an overprotective spouse. To make sure she gets connected to the doctor, Pat says she wants to ask about a certain drug they'd forgotten to mention earlier: Zoplicone, the only drug name that pops into her mind in that second. She says she wants to know if it's safe for Dave to take.

It's a spurious question as Dave certainly doesn't need a sleeping aid (which is what that medication is for) and she had told Dr. Zachary earlier that Dave was refusing all his meds. The nurse says she will page the doctor.

Dr. Zachary phones Pat back at the Lodge. So that the 6 West nurse doesn't get into trouble, Pat says that they forgot to list Zoplicone and the doctor advises that Dave should hold off on that one. Pat then tells him she is very worried about Dave, that he is so much weaker and not answering her questions "on the mark." She is going to add to the report about her concerns but Dr. Zachary interjects tiredly with, "Mrs. Maddocks, bring Dave to 6 West tomorrow morning, as I have asked you to do. Good evening." And the phone goes dead.

There is a knock on their door. It is the Lodge reception desk volunteer with a large commode chair. Pat thanks her for finding it after going to the trouble of phoning her supervisor.

Dave ingests another Imodium. Just minutes pass before his intestines go into contractions and he needs to use the toilet. He willingly allows Pat to set him up on the commode.

She enthuses about how much easier this will be for him, but he's scowling and growls at her, "When are you going to push this thing into the bathroom?"

"But it's a commode, Dave, it *is* a toilet," she says.

But he's insistent, "Please, push this thing, Pat. I can't hold on much longer."

So she does. Her heart breaks. Her clever husband is in deep trouble.

About 10 p.m., there is another knock on the door. It's Ethel, the Lodge's weekend night nurse, a gracious, petite lady from central Asia. She smiles and asks how Dave is doing, as the volunteer receptionist had left a note that the Maddocks had asked for a commode.

"He is not doing well at all," Pat says, her voice cracking with concern. "Please come in. His breathing is just awful."

The nurse sees the rapid rise and fall of Dave's chest as he's sleeping, hears the intensity of the wheezing. She immediately says Dave needs to go to Emergency. Pat tells Nurse Ethel that they had seen Dr. Zachary at the agency earlier that day, that he had said they couldn't admit Dave.

The nurse asks for Dr. Zachary's phone number and she leaves the room to call him. When she returns, she looks embarrassed. She says that the doctor would not change the order, that they are to go to the agency in the morning as previously arranged.

Before the nurse leaves, Pat quietly asks her to give Dave his puffers to help his breathing. He had refused them when Pat had tried to give them to him earlier. But for the nurse, he complies readily. Pat is totally conflicted — furious that he is doing for the nurse what he wouldn't do for her, but grateful that he's taking them.

When they are alone, Pat asks Dave if he'll go to Emergency anyway. She tells him she understands his reluctance. He'd had some really long waits in the ER back home. And this is Vancouver; the newspapers were always reporting horrendous wait times in the ER. Dealing with diarrhea, lying on a gurney parked in a hallway, does not seem like a great option.

Dave is aware that Nurse Ethel phoned Dr. Zachary. He asks Pat what Dr. Zachary said. Pat wants to lie, but she tells him the truth — Dr. Zachary said to come to the agency in the morning.

Dave says, "Then that's what we'll do."

Thankfully, his nightly double dose of Imodium does not trigger another session on the toilet. Pat has elevated the head of his bed. The oxygen is on as high as Dave will allow. He sleeps.

* * * * *

At 3 a.m., the little alarm clock goes off. Pat wakes up Dave to give him more Imodium. But first, he needs to go to the bathroom. Pat gently removes his oxygen cannula and clears the tubing from the carpet. She moves the walker up to his bed, locks the wheels and transfers him from the bed to the little bench seat. He is so weak that she must use her body to prevent him from falling forward and slipping off.

She positions the walker beside the toilet, locks the wheels and starts to transfer him onto the toilet when, suddenly, his body goes stiff in her arms. She's able to get him back down onto the seat of the walker. Terrified that he'll fall and hurt himself on all the hard surfaces, she manages to push him and the walker back on to the carpet, close to his bed. But she can't lift him onto the bed. His head is slammed to one side, his arms and legs are stiff and splayed wide, his heels dug into the carpet. The cord for the emergency bell is on the wall in the bathroom. She backs away from him, her body bent forward, her hands and arms extended so as to be as close to him as she can should he start to slip off the walker. She yanks on the cord and hurries back to him. He isn't breathing.

Almost immediately, Nurse Ethel comes into their room. Both women try to move Dave onto the bed, but they're not strong enough. Instead, they gently ease him onto the carpeted floor. The nurse tries to find his pulse. It isn't there. The nurse asks Pat to increase his oxygen. The nurse starts compressions. She gets his pulse back but it is weak. She quickly calls 911. Within minutes, the paramedics arrive. It is 3:45 a.m., Sunday morning, Day 13 of the trial.

CHAPTER TEN

Final Hours

DECEMBER 4

Within seconds, the room fills with men in blue jumpsuits. They ram the twin beds out of the way, to get more room to work on Dave. Pat instinctively stands back to give them as much space as possible. Two men are kneeling on the floor beside Dave tearing back his nightshirt. Nurse Ethel is reporting to the lead paramedic as Dave lies there unconscious, his pallor alarming. His breathing is shallow and ragged. A clear, wet stain blooms slowly around Dave on the ivory carpet, body fluids draining from his emaciated body.

One of the paramedics urgently asks Pat if there is a Do Not Resuscitate order in place. All the frantic activity ceases. Silence and stillness envelop the room while he waits for her response.

Stunned by the question, Pat manages to say, "Yes." She immediately adds, "It's back home — in Courtenay. But Dave is breathing. I want you to keep trying to help him."

The men in blue quickly unfold a rolling stretcher and throw a brown, pilled blanket from Pat's bed over it. They lift Dave gently. So many hands are on him. His bare, inert body is wrapped, mummy-style, and an oxygen mask is placed over his nose and mouth.

In the few seconds it takes to wheel Dave out of the room, down the hall, out into the cold winter night and into the waiting ambulance, Pat throws on some clothes and is in the passenger seat of the ambulance as the rear doors slam shut.

Minutes later, they are unloading the stretcher onto a dock of one of the bays at the Vancouver General emergency department. Dave is taken to an assessment cubicle and transferred to a thinly padded gurney. They get a saline drip started into his existing IV port. He is awake, cognizant of where he is and who he is with, but he can't answer the doctor's questions about his health history. Pat, through the fog of worry, tells the triage doctor about Dave's participation in the cancer clinical trial of CPX-1 as an outpatient at the cancer agency. The doctor asks for the names of the drugs in the CPX-1 formula. Her head pounds. She just cannot remember; the trial was usually referred to by its initials.

"I have all that information, but it's back at the Lodge," she wails. "I'm sure you can get the drug names from the cancer agency. All that information is on their computers."

"Mrs. Maddocks, the hospitals are not electronically linked," the doctor replies.

"You've got to be kidding!" she blurts out.

The doctor merely shrugs, rolling his eyes.

"Well, the cancer agency has an after-hours phone number," she adds.

"Mrs. Maddocks," he says kindly, "whomever I get at that number isn't going to know anything about this clinical trial. It's 4:30 on a Sunday morning. A doctor certainly isn't going to be there. But I really need to know the names of those drugs. I want you to go back to the Lodge and get those papers."

A little moan escapes her lips. Her eyes tear up as she silently pleads with the doctor to let her stay with Dave. But he insists.

"I really need the names of those drugs, Mrs. Maddocks."

She leaves her position at the foot of the gurney and whispers in Dave's ear that she will be back as quickly as possible, kissing his cheek as she turns to leave. To her relief, Dave seems calm and aware.

Pat rushes out of the cubicle, but gets lost in the maze that is the ER and repeatedly needs to ask for directions, mentally landmarking so that she can easily find her way back. Finally locating the sliding glass doors to the ambulance bays, she asks a paramedic there if the Lodge is to the left or right. With her coat pulled tight around her, she hurries through the darkness, along unfamiliar, frozen sidewalks to the security doors of the Lodge. It takes a long five minutes.

Buzzed in, she grabs the consent form from the top dresser drawer, oblivious to the chaotic mess of their room, and bolts back to the ER. She finds the doctor at the main nursing station and hands him the document.

After just a glance, he says, "As I suspected, Dave is dealing with chemotherapy-induced diarrhea."

"He doesn't have a bacterial infection?" Pat asks, incredulous.

Shaking his head and pointing at the first page, the doctor adds, "No doubt it's this one here. It is such a common side effect with this drug that the illness is specifically named Irinotecan-induced diarrhea. But the good news is that Dave's blood pressure has improved and stabilized. We'll keep the IV going. I've asked the medical department to come and assess him. They should be along shortly."

She goes back to Dave. He seems agitated. He asks her to shift his pillows; he just can't get comfortable on the rock-hard gurney. He lifts his arm, the one not encumbered by the IV tubing, to shield his eyes from the constant glare of the huge overhead flourescent lights. But in doing so, he keeps knocking the oxygen-monitoring clip from his finger. A nurse asks Pat to try and keep his hand still.

Pat tries to protect his eyes with a little tent made from a face-cloth, but this scares Dave; he becomes even more anxious when the fabric brushes his face. And still his gut roils, his every internal organ engaged in painful, spastic efforts to rid itself of the toxic fluids that have built up. His breathing becomes more difficult, his frequent attempts to direct Pat to fix things coming in frustrated rasping gasps.

Hours pass. The nurses bring Pat toast and tea, saying she needs to keep strong, for Dave's sake. About 9:00 a.m., a person from the medical department comes, does a physical assessment on Dave, then orders a lung x-ray.

Pat panics. She doesn't know how Dave can possibly deal with all the jostling involved, with the need to hold his breath. She follows the gurney down the hallway, holding Dave's hand and whispering soothing, tender words while they wait for the x-ray technician. He grips her hand and gazes fearfully into her eyes.

He isn't in the x-ray lab for long, but when they wheel him back to her, his face is a blank mask. Vacantly, he stares straight ahead, doesn't respond at all to her voice. His fingers are still, no longer pleating the flannel sheet as they had been doing constantly for these last long hours.

The porter takes them back to the curtained cubicle. The nurses arrange Dave into a full-sitting position on the gurney to make it easier for him to breathe. His head lolls awkwardly to one side as he dozes fitfully. His feet dangle off the edge, the gurney being too short for his tall frame.

When they are alone once more, she lays her head on his lap and sobs, "Please. Please, Dave. Try harder! Don't leave me!"

The words wrung from her heart shock her. How could she ask for more from this brave man? With virtually no help, for days on end, his valiant body *has* been trying so hard. Pat has watched the emergency ward staff working on Dave and thinks, "He is surrounded by competent, compassionate people. But it is much, much too late."

She rearranges the flannel sheet on his bed and is shocked to discover that his toes and the soles of his feet have turned black. Just last week, she'd noticed his toes under the nails were black, but now it's as though his body is sending a clear message. Pat wonders when exactly that happened. Devastated by the marked change in Dave, she can't stop the tears.

Just then, a young doctor pushes the beige drapes aside

and introduces herself as a renal specialist. This doctor, too, wants to hear about Dave's recent medical history as she uses her stethoscope and fingers to probe his body. Her touch causes Dave's eyes to open but that is the full extent of his response. Pat, clutching the consent form, answers the doctor's every query.

"Mrs. Maddocks," the doctor says, "you know Dave is extremely ill. The acidosis has become—"

Pat interrupts, "Acidosis?"

"Yes," she replies. "Basically, Dave's blood has become acidic. Normally, blood has a neutral pH. A pH of 7.35 is about as low as I like to see it. Dave's is at 7.2."

"What this means," continues the doctor, "is that his blood's pH balance is preventing oxygen from reaching the various parts of his body, which decreases his ability to function. His brain isn't getting enough oxygen, which accounts for his lack of awareness, the blackening of his feet, his poor lung function, his raspy voice and many other problems. I'm particularly concerned about his kidneys. They can't maintain their job of eliminating toxins. His creatinine level of 505 indicates that his kidneys are seriously damaged. I am going to order a catheter to monitor his urine output. We will continue taking blood samples, and then I'll be able to determine if dialysis could be a remedy. I'll get back to you later today."

Pat shudders. To hear that Dave's creatinine level has soared past the dreaded 300 level, that it has doubled yet again from yesterday's ruinous number, shatters her faint hope that Dave can recover.

Pat pulls the privacy curtain closed when the specialist leaves and then slumps into the chair beside Dave's gurney. She removes her glasses with one hand and hides her eyes with the other. Tears leak through her fingers and she brushes them away wearily. Dave remains propped up on pillows, his body somewhere between sleep and unconsciousness. His sheet is rumpled and his feet are uncovered.

Just as she gets up to tuck him in, Dr. Zachary from the cancer agency slides the curtain open. He stands at the end of Dave's gurney, beside the black soles of Dave's feet that are hanging out of the covers, and says stiffly, "Good morning." He looks at Dave but makes no move towards him. He doesn't seem to notice Dave's blackened feet and begins explaining to Pat that he will have a look at Dave's chart and speak with the ER doctor. Then, as he turns to leave, he says, "Mrs. Maddocks, don't worry. We can get Dave over this hump." She so wants to believe him.

About noon, Michele arrives. She had phoned the Lodge inquiring about her dad and was informed he had been taken to emergency. Around the same time, Dave is moved deeper into the crowded maze of the ER. In a tiny cubicle, defined by faded beige draping, there is just room for the gurney. Dave's heart and his oxygen level are no longer being monitored. Pat and Michele sit on vinyl chairs in the cramped corridor. They take turns standing by Dave, who rarely opens his eyes. Taking a quick bathroom break, Pat walks by Dr. Zachary reading a paper at the main nursing station. He mumbles something as she walks by but she doesn't stop. On her return, Michele is being shooed out of Dave's cubicle by a nurse who needs to take a blood sample.

She sits back down beside Pat when the nurse suddenly rushes out, not saying a word. The nurse comes back with a doctor. Pat and Michele exchange worried glances. This is totally unusual. When the nurse comes out a few minutes after the doctor, Pat asks her what is going on.

"We couldn't get a blood sample," she says brusquely. "We had to get it from his groin and I needed a doctor to do that."

It was then that Pat knew Dave's body had shut down. She knew it was over. All day, they'd had trouble getting blood samples. Now it is so difficult they have to give up on accessing his veins and take blood directly from an artery in his groin, a procedure she imagines must be excruciatingly painful.

At 3:00 p.m., the kidney specialist requests a meeting

with Pat and Michele in the family room around the corner. She tells them not one drop of urine has been collected since the catheter was put in, which indicates Dave's kidneys have completely failed. She says that Dave is not a candidate for dialysis, that because his capillaries have shut down and his veins have collapsed, the flushing action of dialysis would not be effective.

The doctor says there is nothing more they can do for Dave, just keep him comfortable and free of pain. She says she expects Dave will not survive much longer. She introduces Michele and Pat to Nurse Florrie who is in charge of palliative care in the ER. The nurse strikes Pat as a good match for the ER environment. She has a calm, gentle demeanour coupled with a clarity and decisiveness that ensures things get done.

Pat was expecting the worst. Any summons they'd ever had to meet with doctors in the past had always resulted in grim news. She knew she was going to hear that Dave was being sentenced to death. Now, she feels empty and numb. She knows it's the end of the fight. Their lives — both of them — are over.

The doctor keeps talking to fill the silence, telling her and Michele about how her own dad had gone through a similar thing and how she doesn't usually share personal information with her patient's families. Michele is listening attentively, but the doctor's words mean nothing to Pat. She is so mired in the grief of losing Dave that she is wholly unable to empathize: this doctor's dad is not Dave. Pat cares only about Dave.

The doctor's words fill the room, but inside Pat's head is silence. Her head is spinning and she feels empty and sore, as if she has just emerged from a boxing ring.

Michele asks if it is possible to have a room with a proper bed so that Dave might have some comfort and privacy. Nurse Florrie is sympathetic but says there are no rooms available. She sees how stricken Pat is and promises to pull out all the stops to find something better. Minutes later she comes back with news that there is an empty cubicle, in a back corner of the ER, with a regular hospital bed and solid panels rather than privacy curtains. It's not much, she says, but better than the tiny space they are in.

Michele and Pat stay in the busy hallway while the nurses move Dave. In such cramped quarters, Pat knows shifting Dave's flaccid frame from the gurney onto a standard hospital bed will be a challenge. Pat is well aware that this effort by the ER staff is a kindly attempt to ease Pat and Michele's distress. Dave himself is way past caring.

Watching the palliative care nurses minister to her husband, Pat can no longer rein in her anger and frustration. The contrast between the aggressive attention Dave is receiving from the VGH ER staff and the casual concern of the cancer agency is painfully obvious.

Pat suddenly realizes that she doesn't know if Dave's body will be required by the clinical trial researchers. She hates herself that such a cold consideration has just popped into her head. She tries to squelch the thought, but she knows that Dave believes strongly in being a part of the search for better cancer treatments. What happens when a trial volunteer dies was not something that was addressed in the consent form. She knows it would be disrespectful to Dave not to follow through.

Pat tentatively asks the question of Nurse Florrie who promptly suggests Pat call the clinical trial doctor to get more information. She is shown to a phone at a nearby nursing station. When she calls the cancer agency's after-hours number, she is put through to Dr. Zachary.

"Dave is dying," Pat says, her voice hard. "The renal specialist says that dialysis is not an option, that nothing more can be done for him."

Dr. Zachary offers conciliatory words, but Pat cuts him off. "Dr. Zachary, I am phoning you to find out if the CPX-1 study will need Dave's body."

There is a lengthy pause and then, with no embellishments, Dr. Zachary says, "No."

The baldness of his answer shocks her.

"Why am I not surprised!" she yells into the phone. "Your damn group had no interest in Dave alive. Why the hell would I think that you might be interested in him when he is dead!"

She slams down the receiver and returns to Dave. In the cubicle, he is lying on his side with the head of the bed just slightly raised. His breathing is laboured and irregular. Pat asks the nurse if the bed is too low, suggesting they raise it a bit more to help his breathing.

"Mrs. Maddocks," says Nurse Florrie, "the doctor has ordered morphine for Dave, to relax him. You can see that his shoulders are raised and extremely tense. That is painful for him and morphine will ease that tension."

"But doesn't morphine make it harder for the lungs to work?" Pat asks.

"It is a low dose and it's important to minimize pain at this point."

Nurse Florrie injects morphine into Dave's IV. Within minutes, his shoulders relax and his breathing seems to improve.

There is only enough room for the bed in this hastily emptied storage space. Michele sits on the left side of the bed near her father. Dave is semi-conscious. Pat sits on the other side of the bed, gazing at his face, gently holding and stroking his limp, thin fingers.

The conversation between Pat and Michele is sporadic, interrupted now and again by Nurse Florrie coming in and checking on Dave, ensuring that he is comfortable. She comes in often, administering another dose of morphine a half hour after the first one. Both Pat and Michele are impressed. Pat can't help commenting to Michele that if Dave had received this much care and attention from the cancer agency, his body would surely have rallied — as it had so many times in the past.

They are reminiscing about all Dave's amazing rebounds from his health crises in the past, when suddenly Dave's head lifts off the pillow and he starts gagging and heaving. Michele quickly pulls him towards her, onto his left side. He starts bleeding from his mouth and nose and Michele tells Pat to go and get a nurse. Within seconds, Pat and the nurse are back with a kidney basin and a fresh sheet and towels. Pat, maneuvering the small bowl, is able to catch some of the fountain of dark red blood that spews from Dave's mouth and nose but most of it goes on the bed and onto Pat's jeans. Dave falls back, lifeless.

Nurse Florrie comes immediately and takes Dave's pulse, but there is nothing to be done. She closes his eyelids and covers the blood with a clean sheet. Dave had signed the Do Not Resuscitate order so there is no rush of medical personnel, no further attempt to help him. It is over. And in that split second, Pat's heart turns to stone.

Jackie, Pat's sister, appears in the doorway, devastated that she has missed the opportunity to say goodbye to Dave. Pat looks at her blankly and says, "Dave died." Jackie is shocked: she didn't know Dave was that sick. The last time she'd seen them was at Dave's birthday at the Japanese restaurant.

She rushes into the room and embraces Michele and Pat. As they stand there weeping, Nurse Florrie cleans Dave's face and removes the IV. She asks them if they would like to stay with Dave for a while. Pat asks Jackie and Michele if they wouldn't mind leaving the room, giving her a few moments alone with Dave.

Pat lies down on the bed with Dave and cuddles into his blanket-covered body. She fondles his silver hair, strokes his big, handsome face and plays with the cleft in his chin. She buries her head in his chest and sobs. She begs him to forgive her for not keeping him safe, for not realizing he was so ill that he was dying, for them not having had a chance to say goodbye to each other.

Even in her grief, she is astonished at how beautiful he looks on his deathbed, his face radiant and peaceful, his long eyelashes splayed on translucent skin.

For more than an hour, she weeps hot tears, pleads incoherently. Finally, she prays: "Eternal rest grant unto Dave, O Lord, and may Your Eternal Light continue to shine upon him. May Dave's soul and the souls of all the creatures You've created, God, through Your mercy, may Dave and they and I live with You, in peace and joy, for ever and ever."

In what feels like only a few minutes, Jackie comes back into the room and tells Pat they must leave. But Pat doesn't want to get up, doesn't want to leave.

Under her sister's steady and sympathetic gaze, she forces herself to get up from the bed. She moves slowly. Her body feels heavy and sluggish. She has to concentrate to move her feet, one in front of the other. She feels as though she has left her life on that hospital bed with Dave. He is dead. She is too.

Then Pat takes a big breath, and goes out into the hallway where the details of the rest of their life are waiting.

CHAPTER 11

Searching

"There are two mistakes one can make on the road to truth … not going all the way, and not starting."

Buddha

After Dave died on Sunday night, December 4, 2005, Pat went back to the Lodge with her sister Jackie. It was unbearable to be there, in that awful room, but it was impossible *not* to be there, desperate as Pat was for the comfort of being among things that belonged to Dave, craving anything that would keep her connected to him. Shocked and exhausted, Pat spent hours talking with Jackie, reliving Dave's week-long battle to survive the lethal dose of CPX-1. Finally, Jackie was able to convince Pat to take a double dose of sleeping pills. It was obvious that Pat needed to rest. Eventually, she fell into a fitful sleep.

The next morning was filled with the activity of packing. The Lodge had made it clear that Pat should settle up and vacate immediately; it is a residence for cancer patients, and now that Dave was deceased, Pat was no longer eligible to stay there. This was no hardship for Pat: Vancouver had become anathema to her. As well, after several back-and-forth phone calls, Pat had booked to meet with a Vancouver funeral parlour — Dave's body needed to be claimed and cared for. In the midst of all this emotional turmoil, Pat was blindsided by a phone call from the clinical trial nurse. Never had Nurse Betsy, of her own volition, initiated a call to the Maddocks and she picked today to express concern! Within seconds of registering who it was, Pat snapped, "You are the last person in the world I want to talk to." Squeezing out a terse "Goodbye," Pat hung up. A short time later, Nurse

Betsy called back. This time, Pat made it clear that she did not want to speak to her. Trying mightily to be courteous, Pat said she would send along a note when she got home to Courtenay.

Within minutes the phone rang again. It was Dr. Xavier! Pat was totally incapable of listening to the banalities emanating from this man. Pat interrupted his spiel. Between clenched teeth, she ground out that she couldn't talk to him and ended the call with a promise that she would respond later, in writing.

Michele arrived at the Lodge just as Pat and her sister were getting ready to leave to meet the funeral director. Michele had just come from the BCCA clinical trials department, where she had discussed Dave's ordeal and the fact that Pat was critical of the quality and quantity of care that Dave had received from the Phase I team. She reported that the medical staff insisted that a doctor's summary, filed by Dr. Xavier, stated that on the Friday, December 2, Dave had looked better.

"Looked better — on Friday — ridiculous!" Pat blurted. "God, how I wish Dave *had* been better on Friday! But why would Dr. Xavier write that when I told him that the Imodium just wasn't working. And just before that, I'd told the trial nurse that Dave was way too sick to have the next infusion on Tuesday."

At that moment, honouring Dave's wishes to have his body cremated was uppermost in Pat's mind and she shrugged off Michele's report. That discrepancy was one of many that would come back to haunt her in the days and months to come.

When she got back home to Courtenay, accompanied by Jackie and Michele, the three women set to work notifying friends and family of Dave's death, making phone calls, arranging for obituaries, printing out and mailing memoriam cards. But Pat also got on the Internet and looked up chemotherapy-induced diarrhea. What she found on the BCCA website astounded her. And in that moment, all her doubts about the quality of care meted out to her husband during the Phase I trial gelled into an absolute conviction that Dave's Phase I "care package" certainly had not included even the standard crisis remedies given to regular cancer patients. Consent form rhetoric aside, Dave's recruitment into the Phase I trial changed his status from "cancer patient" to "human subject." A patient does not expect to be deliberately put in harm's way by their doctor, but that is the constant reality of being a human subject in a Phase I trial.

At her kitchen table, looking out over the snowy fields, Pat went through the logs she had so carefully kept during the clinical trial. She added notes and details that she didn't want to forget. Pat phoned the manager of the Lodge and asked her if she would access Dave's medical records — explaining that she needed to better understand what had happened to Dave. The manager said she could do that, but it would be quicker for Pat to ask BCCA directly. As Dave's executor, she said, his records belonged to her.[1]

Pat immediately called the cancer agency and they faxed the required form to Pat's family lawyer, as her signature would need to be notarized. Her lawyer then couriered the completed application back to the agency.

Michele was equally appalled by the traumatic ending of her father's life. She and Pat decided together that they would not play the blame game but would concentrate, instead, on improving care for future Phase I volunteers at BCCA, so they might avoid the grizzly outcome experienced by Dave. They began to design a Patient Grid Sheet that would enable Phase I volunteers to systematically track their own health changes.

On December 14, Pat wrote her first complaint letter to BCCA, sending it to every individual and organization connected medically with Dave's trial.

"It is with a heaviness of heart and a sense of futility that I attempt to compose this letter. Truly, I am trying to keep my anger and disappointment out of this missive for I know

1. Pat hadn't known that a patient's entire medical record is the real property of the patient. When she'd asked for and had been given Dave's lab reports, she thought it was just a courtesy.

that you will not be responsive to emotion. Please, dismiss my feelings where they break through and just digest the facts.

"My daughter, a PAR nurse, is urging me to communicate with you and your associates while the events that led to my husband's death are still fresh — in your minds and charts. She seems to think that your organization is capable of being able to change its 'modus operandi' from evaluating pages of numbers generated by lab tests to assessing 'head to toe' the actual person. My faith in your capabilities has been, and remains, severely shaken. But to give my daughter some peace, I will, again, try to get you people to comprehend the agony that David endured — in an effort to inspire you to change your ways.

"Specifically, my concern is the lack of effective patient monitoring procedures in the Phase I trial of CPX-1. My dread is that other patients will be exposed to and expire from BCCA's failure to perform the due diligence required to fulfill the promises that it makes to all trial participants."

In her letter, Pat asked for clarification of a number of things. She asked for the exact cause of Dave's death, and whether the scientific protocol governing the conduct of the CPX-1 trial was comprehensive enough. She wanted to know why Imodium was the only remedy offered to Dave when the standard response for controlling severe diarrhea, as indicated on BCCA's own website, is 24-hour hydration and hospitalization, as well as intervention with the drug Octreatide. But mainly, she questioned whether the Phase I researchers had effective methods in place to fulfill the written promises they'd made to Dave in the Subject Information and Consent Form, promises such as: "your safety is our primary concern; your doctor will watch you closely and respond rapidly; all care will be taken ..."

Pat had several concrete suggestions for improving care. She wrote that Phase I volunteers should wear a patient identification bracelet that would list the drugs being tested and the agency contact information. As well, each Phase I volunteer should keep a daily record of their health status. This record sheet should then be read diligently and in a timely manner by agency researchers and by the contract research organization.[2] As well, this record sheet should then become part of the official Patient Record. Pat requested that the cancer agency physically show her what changes would be made to effect better care of Phase I volunteers as she now had no confidence in either their spoken or written guarantees.

Her letter concluded: "I ask you, politely, to please respond to my concerns in a timely manner. Possibly, David's gruesome death will motivate you to re-examine your methods of patient assessment. Yes, I know David would have died anyway — so will you, so will I. I know he couldn't have been saved. But, dear God, could he not have been spared such an ignominious and crisis-ridden exit? Please, see if you can change something, anything, so that more already heavily burdened souls are not pitched into the agony that was David's last few days."

Pat received a telephone reply from Dr. Susan O'Reilly, BCCA's VP of Cancer Care and Director of Clinical Trials. Condolences expressed, Dr. O'Reilly offered to meet with Pat and her family. Pat agreed that maybe later a meeting could be useful, but she wanted a written response to her letter. Dr. O'Reilly assured her she was already working on generating a report.

The College of Nurses also verbally acknowledged Pat's concerns about the lack of patient advocacy displayed by BCCA's Nurse Betsy and its Medical Daycare department. The College forwarded a copy of the complaint package to the Head of Nursing Practice at BCCA.

The College of Physicians and Surgeons of British Columbia responded as well, asking Pat to continue to communicate with BCCA, but urging her to get back to the College should that route prove unsuccessful.

---

2. A Contract Research Organization or CRO is a company contracted by the sponsor of a clinical trial to collect and manage the scientific data that results from the copious lab tests performed on clinical trial subjects. In Dave's CPX-1 trial, the sponsor — Celator Pharmaceuticals — hired PRA International. This particular CRO is associated with clinical trials in 85 countries over six continents and has been in operation for over 30 years.

The Lodge's response was gratifyingly sincere. They immediately posted, on the back of each bedroom door, a lengthy list of all the health care aids available to residents — including commodes and nutritionally fortified drinks.

On January 3, 2006, Pat received Dave's Patient Record.[3] Reading through it, she was astounded by the variations between what was on the pages and what she remembered from that terrible week of just one month ago. There was so much that wasn't noted about the communications between the Maddocks and BCCA regarding Dave's ever-worsening situation.

The clinical trial nurse's assessment record was a single, double-sided page with widely spaced lines haphazardly scrawled in a loopy longhand. The front of the sheet was all about the steps taken to recruit Dave. Two-thirds of the back page chronicled just three days of Dave's involvement with the CPX-1 trial. Nurse Betsy hadn't written anything about how she had advised Dave to take over-the-counter medications, or her orders to reduce prescribed ones. She didn't note that Dave was thinking of forgoing the next dose of CPX-1, nor that on the next day he had refused to continue with the trial because he was just too sick. The remaining third of the back page was devoted to who was notified of Dave's death.

The Doctor's Summary from the November 17 meeting when Dave and Pat had signed the Subject Information and Consent Form stated, "He [Dave] is aware that treatment is palliative and the hope is to control the disease and improve quality of life."[4] Pat wondered if Dr. Timothy had even read the consent form that he had co-signed, especially the part

3. The more than three-week wait was due to BCCA policy, according to their receptionist. If a request for a Patient Record arrives with a lawyer's letterhead, then the Record must be vetted by a supervisor before being released.

4. In separate conversations with a professor of oncology at the University of Sydney and with a noted genetic biologist, I commented that the scant literature available on these experiments says there is a possibility that 4 percent of Phase 1 cancer clinical trial subjects will experience improvement. Both these gentlemen immediately assured me that percentage number is much too high; that the rate is, in fact, significantly lower.

that stated that "no patient benefit is expected." This doctor's comment was even more amazing to Pat, for when she had earlier asked Dr. Xavier if the proffered experiment was considered to be palliative chemotherapy, she had been told, firmly and succinctly, "No."

A Doctor's Summary, authored by Dr. Xavier, dated Friday, December 2, said, "Clinically he looks clearly better than yesterday." And yet, there was no Doctor's Summary dated December 1 with which a comparison could be drawn. To Pat that meant that the December 2 observation was a conclusion reached strictly from assessments of lab reports.

A Doctor's Summary from Dr. Zachary for Saturday, December 3 said, "He had 2+ edema peripherally as he had done for the last two weeks." But the Doctor's Summary from Tuesday, November 29, written by Dr. Xavier, stated there was "No peripheral edema."[5] The lab report from Dave's blood samples taken on that same morning reported a creatinine level of 288 but Pat thought they had been told the value was 250.

Still, Pat decided to set aside these apparent inconsistencies in Dave's medical records and wait for a response to her complaint letter. One evening, a week after receiving Dave's Patient Record, she got another call from Dr. O'Reilly. Surprised, Pat listened as the doctor apologized for calling so late.

Dr. O'Reilly explained that she had just finished meeting with Dr. Joseph Connors, chairman of the UBC–BCCA Research Ethics Board. She enthused that in addition to a report that would be forthcoming from the two of them, there would be a Mortality and Morbidity Review from a committee that Dr. O'Reilly had convened. Dr. O'Reilly said that because Dave had actually died at VGH, his death was not a BCCA issue. Still, a cancer agency panel, chaired by a Dr.

5. Doctors' summaries, as well as all test results, are the property of the patient. Several days can elapse before doctors' summaries are transcribed and actually become part of the Patient Record.

Judith Pike, would look into the management of Dave's care prior to his demise.

Pat, holding her temper in check, calmly asked the doctor not to telephone anymore, but to make contact either by letter or email. She was incensed, feeling that the spokesperson for the researchers was acting like she was doing a favour for the Maddocks family by conducting these investigations — like they were bestowing some sort of grand honour on Dave. Dr. O'Reilly's call precipitated Pat's deciding to write directly to Dr. Simon Sutcliffe, President of the BCCA, to draw his attention to points in Dave's Patient Record that she felt needed clarification.

That done, Pat wrote again to Dr. Connors and asked him if it was naive of the Maddocks family to expect the Ethics Board to focus on the Board's raison d'être — namely the protection of the physical and mental well-being of human subjects enrolled in clinical trials. Pat again asked the Ethics Board whether the rules for conducting a Phase I trial at BCCA, rules established by the Ethics Board, were truly effective. Dr. Connors responded personally to this letter, assuring Pat that he would issue a report separate from that of the VP of Cancer Care.

To Pat, Dr. O'Reilly's nine-page report, issued on February 17, 2006, was a lengthy non-event. A lot of ink was dedicated to rehashing Dave's medical history prior to the trial, followed by a *Reader's Digest* version of the doctors' summaries penned by Dr. Xavier and Dr. Zachary.

"Mr. Maddocks died from renal failure due to fluid loss from vomiting and diarrhea related to his treatment[6] with the

6. Dave did not receive "treatment with ... CPX-1"; he underwent exposure to CPX-1. The end purpose of medical treatment is beneficial; the end purpose of the Phase 1 experimental process is noxious. Thus it is a misnomer to use the word "treatment" in referring to a stratagem that seeks to determine lethality. The test drug CPX-1 was designed to have an impact on colon cancer. In Dave's case, the likelihood of his esophageal and liver cancer being remedied was next to zero. In a Phase 1 trial, the subject's cancer is not necessarily matched up to the test product's area of possible usefulness; just a body, dying of cancer but with functioning major organs, is required.

experimental drug CPX-1," wrote Dr. O'Reilly.

Some obvious comments were proffered, such as "Mr. Maddocks should have been admitted to hospital on Saturday December 3 for continuous intravenous hydration and bicarbonate." And if that was not possible, then "the patient should have been transferred to VGH emergency."

Dr. O'Reilly noted that "Dr. Zachary also notified Dr. Yvonne, the medical oncology staff member on call, of the patient's clinical status and, at that time, Dr. Zachary and Dr. Yvonne felt that the management plan was appropriate." And further along in her letter, "Dr. Zachary saw Mr. Maddocks twice in the course of the late morning and afternoon of Dec. 4/05 and he also contacted Dr. Yvonne to advise her of the deterioration in Mr. Maddocks' condition. Dr. Yvonne did not see Mr. Maddocks during the weekend of December 3 or 4."

The existence of a third possible resource for Dave, a Dr. Yvonne, had never been communicated to Dave and Pat. Dr. O'Reilly also stated, "Everyone is well aware of our usual standard that the emergency room physician is always notified and provided clinical information regarding any patient being transferred."

Dr. O'Reilly explained the inability of doctors to access patient data between institutions by saying that there was a lack of "privacy agreements between the five regional health authorities and the Provincial Health Service Authority."[7]

In her report, Dr. O'Reilly wrote, "The important issue in Mr. Maddocks' case is that Mrs. Maddocks would have been spared some distress and concern regarding the transfer of information had Dr. Zachary been proactive in telephoning the emergency physician to advise him of Mr. Maddocks' situation."

Pat suspected that Dr. O'Reilly was being somewhat obtuse in stating that, of all the hardships that she and Dave

---

7. The Provincial Health Service Authority (PHSA) is responsible for governing medical facilities that are used by all of the province's population, not for a specific region as is the case with the other five health authorities. Dr. O'Reilly's comment indicated that a possible turf war existed between these organizations.

had endured, Dr. Zachary's failure to phone the Vancouver General Hospital's ER was "the important issue in Mr. Maddocks' case."

The only real actions undertaken to improve the monitoring of Phase I subjects were noted under the heading of Recommendations for Improvements. Apparently Dr. O'Reilly had met with both medical oncologists and residents and reviewed the existing codes of patient care. The sum total of improvements to monitoring Phase I volunteers was minor revisions that felt more cosmetic than substantive. The status quo was unchanged.

Dr. O'Reilly further stated that "we did not achieve the optimal care and support that we wish to provide." But she added, "I am of the opinion that reasonable efforts were made in the care of Mr. Maddocks on the weekend of December 3 and 4."

Dr. O'Reilly also concluded that the monitoring and management of Mr. Maddocks "was appropriate for his situation between Tuesday, November 29 and Friday, December 2."

Despite stating that Dave's care had been "reasonable" and "appropriate," Dr. O'Reilly wrote, "On behalf of the Medical Oncology staff at the Vancouver Cancer Centre and the British Columbia Cancer Agency, we would like to offer our sincere apologies for not achieving the level of care that you and Mr. Maddocks anticipated. We offer you our sincere regrets that Mr. Maddocks had such a miserable experience in the last few days of his life."

Dr. O'Reilly's choice of words rankled. Of course, Pat and Dave had "anticipated" that Dave would receive "optimal" care — that anticipation was a direct result of their dialogues with BCCA researchers and with the wording of the consent form. A thinking human being could agree to endure the physical and mental rigours of a clinical trial, especially a Phase I, *only* if they believed that they would be well looked after. "Anticipated" implied to Pat that she and Dave had been unrealistic in their expectation that BCCA researchers would fulfill their promises of careful attention made in the consent form. And "miserable experience"? Pat had heard of a miserable cold, but she didn't think dehydrating to death was akin to dealing with a runny nose.

Dr. O'Reilly ended her report with a renewed invitation to the Maddocks family to meet with herself and Dr. Connors.

Pat wanted to be mollified by these pages of assurances that researchers would communicate more effectively with one another, that they would, henceforth, adhere to established protocols.

Apparently, communication practices between doctors had been tweaked. However, Pat's call for changes to communication practices between the Phase I team and its *test subjects* was not addressed. This, in Pat's mind, was the underlying and systematic failure, the real cause of Dave's "miserable experience." Among Dr. O'Reilly's Recommendations for Improvements was the sentence, "I have asked the Phase I team medical staff to notify both the on-call resident and staff oncologists if they are concerned about an outpatient." The pivotal words "if they are concerned" nailed down the problems that Dave and Pat had battled. Pat considered that the Phase I team was not concerned about Dave's severe adverse events because the events had not been noted and thus crucial calls were not made. Her point was that watching Dave very closely had not occurred. The report did not specify any measures aimed at the better monitoring of Phase I subjects so that medical staff would be motivated to be concerned, concerned enough to act — to "respond rapidly" as the consent form promised.[8]

Less than a week later, on February 21, 2006, UBC–BCCA Research Ethics Board Chairman Dr. Joseph Connors issued

8. The National Cancer Institute website thoroughly explains the Phase 1 clinical trial process. Under "Information Sources for Grading AEs (adverse events)," it encourages the use of Patient Diary Reports. Under the heading History and Physical Exam: "It has been demonstrated that AEs will not be identified unless appropriate questions are asked and necessary examinations performed. It is necessary to develop interviewing techniques to elicit important AE information from patients."

his own review. "Having established that the proper procedures for the conduct of phase I testing are already in place, I examined the series of events surrounding your husband's death to determine if these procedures were adequately applied and if further changes in these procedures should be made. These specific details are thoroughly discussed in Dr. O'Reilly's report.[9] Her findings concerning the specific actions of individual physicians involved are described there. I will not repeat them. My own finding is that the standard procedures in place for phase I trial subjects were not fully followed." Dr. Connors continued, "In particular, notification of phase I on-call study doctor and early hospitalization, as recommended by the phase I program, were not performed."

Dr. Connors went on to explain his position by stating, "My role as the Research Ethics Board Chair is not to make a judgment about the medical care that your husband received. It is, rather, to determine if there is any aspect of the phase I program that should be changed. My finding is that the deficiency in this case was not with the procedures that are in place, but rather that these procedures were not always followed. In particular, I would focus on the communication between the medical staff looking after your husband on that weekend and the phase I program study doctors. It is Dr. O'Reilly's responsibility to take action to correct this problem with communication."

Finally an acknowledgement that pivotal mistakes were made. Now, according to the Ethics Board Chair, it was up to Dr. O'Reilly to find ways to get her staff to do what they were supposed to do. But, again, the spotlight was put on the medical practitioners when what was lacking was focus on the human being used as a test subject.

Pat asked Dr. O'Reilly for the Morbidity and Mortality Report (MMR). Despite the doctor's earlier assurances that the

9. Dr. Connors refers earlier in his letter to "Dr. O'Reilly's review of these events as summarized to you in her letter of 09 February 2006." The report from Dr. O'Reilly that Pat received was dated February 17, 2006.

Maddocks family would receive a copy, however, Pat was now informed it was not legally possible for her to have it even though Dr. O'Reilly claimed that BCCA truly wanted Pat to have it.[10]

Her faith in Dr. O'Reilly and her agency further eroded, Pat decided to get in touch with Celator Pharmaceuticals, the sponsor of the CPX-1 trial. She wanted a guarantee that Phase I volunteers would be fully informed, not just initially but continuously throughout the trial, and she wanted to change the wording of the consent form to specifically state that there was *a risk of death* in place of the medical euphemism of "life-threatening side effects are possible."

Dr. Andrew Janoff, CEO of Celator, emailed Pat that the consent form was not written by Celator but was a research industry standard personalized by each contracted medical institution.[11] He was adamant that he and his company were fully supportive of Pat's efforts to improve care for Phase I volunteers and encouraged her to contact him if he could be of assistance.

He volunteered copies of Dave's CIOMS form, paperwork she had never seen before as it had not been included in Dave's Patient Record.[12] Dr. Janoff told Pat that BCCA had filed four different versions of Dave's form. In all the forms, including the final one dated March 7, 2006, Pat again found inaccuracies, mainly in specifics of Dave's care management and the dates when events occurred.

---

10. Under Section 51 of the BC *Evidence Act*, any MMR / Q & A report is "not available to members of the public, patients or lawyers — to allow for quality improvement without risk to organizations or individuals."

11. The "boilerplate" version can be found, with diligence, on the National Cancer Institute (NCI) website.

12. CIOMS stands for Council for International Organizations of Medical Sciences, a think-tank associated with WHO and UNESCO. In any clinical trial, when a severe adverse event (SAE) occurs, the principal investigator (PI) responsible for the day-to-day operations must fill out a form designed by the CIOMS. The completed form is filed with the Therapeutic Products Directorate of Health Canada (HC). When a subject dies, the form must be filed within seven working days. HC receives these forms and files them; the information is available to HC and to that trial's research team. HC processed 100 CIOMS forms each day in 2006 and 450 to 500 CIOMS forms each day in 2010.

The arrival of Dave's CIOMS form was a "light bulb" moment for Pat. Until then, she had been solely concerned with improving the monitoring of Phase I human subjects at BCCA. As so often happens in life, she'd lost sight of the "forest" — the initial reason *why* Dave had volunteered for the CPX-1 trial; namely, to further cancer research. She had become fixated on the "trees," what had happened to Dave. In the reports she'd received, communication between doctors had been identified as defective but she now worried that the systems in place to distribute the data collected from Phase I volunteers to the entire research community might not have functioned smoothly either. She hadn't given a single thought to just how such data is disseminated.

With the discovery of these CIOMS forms, the implications were even more serious; there was a much wider database possibly tainted by wrong information. Pat fired off a letter to the Chief Scientist at Health Canada (HC) pointing out where the CIOMS information was incorrect and asking for an audit.

Health Canada's Director General, Omer Boudreau, replied, "we do not regulate the practice of medicine. This falls to the purview of provincial authorities, in your case of the College of Physicians and Surgeons of British Columbia. We can investigate fraud and related matters through Health Canada's Health Products and Food Branch Inspectorate, but from your letter I understand that your complaints are related to the medical care of your husband." Further, he mentioned that Dr. Connors' review had said there was no misconduct in the Ethics Board's handling of this clinical trial and Health Canada could find no fault with the CIOMS forms. "Unfortunately," wrote Mr. Boudreau, "you are now very much aware of the risks of participating in medical research trials. We regret your distress."

Pat's request for an audit was denied.[13] The competence of the "practice of medicine" during a Phase I clinical trial

---

13. Annually, less than 2 percent of institutions conducting clinical trials are audited by HC, due to a lack of inspectors.

is crucial to obtaining valid observations and data. It seemed strange that HC was divorced from regulating the personnel responsible for the accuracy of the information by which new drugs attain HC's approval. Dave, in the consent form, had been obliged to agree that his trial data could "be sent to Health Canada (because it oversees the use of drugs in this country)." Mr. Boudreau's assertion, though, was that HC has no authority over those who administer these drugs.

In March of 2006, after Dr. O'Reilly had informed Pat that the MMR Report could not legally be released to the Maddocks family, she again offered to arrange for the family to meet with any senior member of the BCCA. Dr. O'Reilly was scheduled to be out of the country for some weeks, so Pat, Michele and Jackie arranged to meet with Dr. O'Reilly and Dr. Connors on April 18, 2006.

Pat had attempted to set up a separate family meeting with Dr. Connors and also one with the BCCA Head of Nursing Practice, but was told by their secretaries that Dr. Connors would be joining their meeting with Dr. O'Reilly and that the Head of Nursing was not available at all.

On Friday, April 7, Pat had a surprise telephone call from Dr. O'Reilly. She wanted to know what Pat and her family intended to discuss at the upcoming meeting and casually cautioned Pat not to bring a lawyer. Pat assured the doctor that she and her family were working on an agenda, one that would focus entirely on ways to improve monitoring of Phase I volunteers, and that she would email it around the following week. Dr. O'Reilly asked Pat if there was anything else she wanted to know — Pat had previously emailed a request for specifics on BCCA policy. Pat then mentioned that she was disappointed that the Head of Nursing Practice had declined to meet with the Maddocks family. Dr. O'Reilly informed Pat that it was she, Dr. O'Reilly, who had decided such a meeting would not be helpful. Then the doctor asked why Pat had made an inquiry about doctors' billings to the BCCA accounting department.

Pat explained that she had previously asked the Medical Services Plan of B.C. for that information but was eventually told that MSP doesn't pay Phase I doctors. Dr. O'Reilly replied that she paid them; that research doctors are paid a flat fee and thus it wasn't necessary to track their activities. The doctor then asked Pat why she wanted to know. Pat said that after reading the doctors' summaries, she felt that too much emphasis was placed on interpreting lab reports and not enough hands-on attention was given to the actual patient. Pat cited the Doctor's Summary of December 2 as an example. Dr. O'Reilly had the specific report at hand and she read Pat the entire, but short, summary filed by Dr. Xavier for that day. Pat, pointing out that the report said "clinically" Dave appeared "better," suggested that the report was a summarization of lab reports from Dec. I and 2. Dr. O'Reilly assured Pat that "clinically" meant that the doctor had attended Dave. Noting that no time or location had been specified, Pat asked Dr. O'Reilly to confirm those details with Dr. Xavier, which the doctor agreed to do.

On April 11, 2006, Dr. O'Reilly emailed: "I spoke to Dr. Xavier re the location where he saw Mr. Maddocks on December 2. It was in Medical Daycare, in the afternoon, between 3:00 and 3:30. Dr. Xavier recollects you were in the room at the same time."

Pat emailed back saying she had no recollection of that and asked Dr. O'Reilly to check with the nurses and cleaning staff on the sixth floor.

The next day, Dr. O'Reilly responded. "Dr. Xavier's times are very approximate. He not only saw Mr. Maddocks but documented it clearly, so I'm not pursuing this further."

Pat went ahead with the meeting April 18 between her family and Dr. O'Reilly and Dr. Connors. She desperately wanted to see monitoring and management improve for future Phase I volunteers. Pat suggested that all doctors' summations include information about when and where a doctor's consultation with a human subject takes place. She pointed out that such basic details are necessary to guarantee the integrity of any summary and could help towards achieving the scientific community and general public's call for transparency and accountability in pharmaceutical research.

She also suggested that the agency and the Lodge develop a closer working relationship. Pat said that the Lodge's Unusual Incident Report,[14] which Pat had obtained and sent to the cancer agency's management, highlighted a need for re-evaluation of the agency's rapport with that vital service to cancer consumers.[15]

Dr. O'Reilly said Pat's suggestion that a member of the Phase I research team telephone and speak directly to the Phase I volunteer at least three times a week throughout the subject's involvement with a trial would be given consideration, as would her suggestion to change the wording on the consent form to read "risk of death," instead of the current medical euphemism "life threatening."

At one point in the meeting, Pat's sister Jackie, in a discussion about patient monitoring, said, "When Dave donated his body to science, he —"

"Why, he did no such thing!" interrupted Dr. O'Reilly. "What are you talking about?"

Stunned by the outburst, Jackie coldly continued, "Madame, Dave *did* donate his *living* body to science. Your lack of appreciation of that gift explains why Dave and Pat have been treated so shabbily."

The meeting lasted two hours. Dr. Connors promised to respond to the points brought out in the meeting by letter,

14. Jackie, a former nurse, had informed Pat that an Unusual Incident Report is required from medical staff when something out-of-the-ordinary occurs during a shift. An institution will not inform you of this documentation and you must go through legal hoops to obtain it. In March of 2006, the Lodge's lawyer released this report filed by Night Nurse Ethel. She stated that she informed Dr. Zachary immediately of Dave's transfer by ambulance to the ER at VGH. Pat had forwarded that report to Dr. O'Reilly and the supervisor of resident doctors at BCCA.

15. "Cancer consumer" is the phrase used by Breast Cancer Action Group NSW (Australia) to refer to people affected by cancer.

in three weeks. But Dr. O'Reilly immediately countermanded him, saying it would take three months. Pat left with few expectations and a growing sense of disappointment.

The next day, Pat and Jackie had a cordial meeting with Dr. Sutcliffe, president of BCCA. He agreed that his agency should inform its patients that their medical records are not available between institutions.[16] He said it was the provincial government's Privacy Commissioner's Office, not the medical institutions, that was holding up the electronic integration of patient records.[17] He assured Pat and Jackie that both he and the CEO of the Provincial Health Services Authority (PHSA) were keen to provide identification bracelets or wallet cards to outpatient volunteers in Phase I trials.

Two days later, after a renewed request to Dr. O'Reilly, Pat met with the Head of Nursing Practice at BCCA. She listened as Pat expressed her family's concern that the nursing routine at the agency's Medical Daycare had not included any documented observations of Dave's clinical condition — either before, during or after he had mini sessions of hydration. Pat also wanted the role of the clinical trial nurse to be expanded, pointing out that the person filling that position in a Phase I team must be more involved, more of an advocate for the Phase I volunteer. Pat was hopeful leaving that meeting. The Head of Nursing seemed to understand her family's concerns. Pat thought they had now found someone who could change policy and was willing to do it. The Head of Nursing admitted that it would take more than seven months to educate staff and to get any new routines working smoothly, but Pat believed change was possible.

---

16. The parents of patients managed by BC Children's Hospital are provided the tools to keep an at-home, up-to-date medical file on their child. Children's Hospital encourages parents to take this file to all doctor's consultations and whenever they are traveling — exactly because there is no electronic transfer of patient information between medical institutions. BCCA and Children's are governed by the same health authority — PHSA. Strangely, a patient's prescription drug history can be easily accessed from anywhere in the province, but not their medical records.

17. Banks, casinos and retail enterprises of every ilk have solved the electronic technology and privacy issues that seem to have befuddled the B.C. government.

Four months later, a succinct letter arrived, authored by Dr. O'Reilly and also signed by both Dr. Connors and Dr. Sutcliffe. Dr. O'Reilly wrote that the Head of Nursing was reviewing guidelines for improved nursing documentation of patients. She said the revised consent forms would now include the words "might even cause death." The possibility of inter-hospital electronic sharing of patient records was snarled indefinitely, she wrote, due to inadequate technology and privacy issues, but BCCA and PHSA were committed to establishing such a system.

In Pat's reply, she asked for a sample of the identification bracelets that Dr. Sutcliffe had said would be no problem to implement. She also asked for a copy of the revised consent form. But she never received an answer to her letter, nor to any continued efforts on her part to communicate. All dialogue ceased. They were, it seemed, no longer willing to talk to her.

Feeling that all her options were exhausted, Pat wrote a formal letter of complaint to the College of Physicians and Surgeons of British Columbia, dated November 30, 2006. In it, she cited Dr. Xavier for "not providing the leadership required for the effective management of the severe side effects of CPX-1 exhibited by Mr. Maddocks for a full five days."[18]

Pat then documented the number of times she'd contacted the Phase I team, nurse and doctors. They had never once called to see how Dave was doing. "During my daily, sometimes three or four, conversations in person and by phone with the trial nurse and Dr. Xavier, we were given the impression that we must just try harder to deal with our problems, that what Dave was experiencing was just the norm for chemotherapy."

Pat asked the College to review Dr. Zachary's handling of Dave's decline. To support her request, she quoted from Dr. O'Reilly's February 17, 2005, report: "On Saturday, his situation had clearly deteriorated over the preceding night. He was having more diarrhea, he was not taking fluids

18. Only complaints against specific doctors are heard by the College.

orally, and not only was his creatinine rising steeply, he was developing metabolic abnormalities in his blood tests indicating serious deterioration. Despite Dr. Zachary's clinical impression that the patient's condition was relatively stable and the administration of intravenous fluids in Daycare was appropriate, both Mr. Maddocks' comfort and overall clinical management would have been best delivered on an in-patient basis on December 3."

Pat also cited Dr. Yvonne in her complaint letter to the College. Dr. O'Reilly's report of February 17 had stated, "Although Dr. Zachary communicated with Dr. Yvonne, the staff doctor on call for medical oncology, who agreed with the management plan, they did not take the step of notifying Phase I team doctors conducting the clinical trial on which he had been enrolled."

Pat backed up her complaints by including the information that "Researchers were made aware by Celator, the test drug's sponsor, that 'careful attention should be paid to managing diarrhea and vomiting.'"[19] She also submitted her own documentation of Dave's Diarrhea and Medication Incidences to substantiate that, for five days, Mr. Maddocks, virtually on his own, dealt with Level 3 and 4 chemotherapy-induced diarrhea.[20] She drew the College's attention to the fact that the BCCA's own care guidelines, provided on their website, call for immediate hospitalization and 24-hour hydration with the use of Octreatide for any cancer patient dealing with severe side effects of chemotherapy-induced diarrhea.

"Dave's last six days," she wrote, "were a ghastly finale for a guy who made the donation of the remaining days of his life to help future cancer patients."

The College advised Pat to have patience, as each doctor had

19. Quote from the sponsor generated investigator's brochure (IB), with which all researchers attached to the CPX-1 study were supposed to be familiar. The IB is a document that every clinical trial must have available and, with effort, can be obtained by the human subject enrolled in the trial.

20. Level 5 chemotherapy-induced diarrhea is death.

to be informed of her accusations, at which point they would be required to submit a written rebuttal, and that it would be a minimum of six months before the review by the College would be completed. Early in 2007, Pat was told the process might take longer, since they couldn't find Dr. Zachary. That was the last straw.

PLAN B

All through the long, torturous hours that Pat spent trying to make sense of the calamity that had befallen Dave, she had one small piece of solace — if the powers-that-be would not give her proof that the monitoring of Phase I volunteers was substantially improved, she would take them to court.

The consent form she and Dave had signed specifically stated, "You do not waive any of your legal rights for compensation by signing this form."

After consulting a couple of Vancouver medical malpractice lawyers, she found out there was a two-year window in which she could launch a civil lawsuit. That window would close December 4, 2007 — the second anniversary of Dave's death.

She discovered that civil court is not about spearheading change or obtaining justice, it is about money — the dollar value of the damages done to the complainant. She found out that no one could be held accountable for what Dave had endured because Dave was dead and, thus, had no need for compensation. She learned that in civil court, a retired person or a child is usually worth nothing; if a Canadian is not earning wages, they have no value.[21] The only basis for a lawsuit was the damage that had been done to *her*!

Pat also found out that she had played "the game" all wrong. To impress the court, immediately upon Dave's death she should have established a medical record of stress and trauma she

21. Some Canadians have a cultural tradition of children supporting their aged parents. In specific cases, if that can be proven to be the norm, then prorated, projected lost income due to the death or injury of the child might be awarded. *Heidi Dawn Klompas: Missed Opportunities* by Catherine S. Adamson addresses this issue.

suffered due to the circumstances surrounding Dave's death. It would have been smarter to have been under psychiatric care and medicated than striving to function independently.

Pat looked into taking the whole mess to the Provincial Ombudsman, but she found out that this office does not get involved with medical complaints.

In the spring of 2007, she did participate in the BC Government's Conversation on Health, as a member of a panel discussing the frustrations people had encountered in the healthcare system. It was a fortuitous decision. At a session in Campbell River, Pat met Eliska, a European woman who had taken on the Alberta healthcare system seeking justice for her adult son who was irreversibly brain injured as the result of medical error. Eliska knew exactly what Pat was coping with and was eager to share her hard-earned expertise. When Pat confided to Eliska that the College was reviewing Dave's case, Eliska had some excellent advice. "Don't get your hopes up that the College will address the issue of test subject monitoring. After all, it is the doctors' own organization and their natural inclination is to protect their own members."

"Actually, if I can fully understand what happened to Dave then maybe our efforts to improve how clinical trial volunteers are cared for will be more effective," Pat replied.

"If you want that, then you are going to want to read the doctors' rebuttal letters. The College will not offer them to you. But you can get them," Eliska said. "Here's what you do. When you get their review, write back and politely refuse to accept their conclusions. You'll have to have a valid reason but I assure you, that part will be easy. At the same time, ask for copies of the doctors' letters. There'll be more paperwork, but you can get those letters."

Pat was grateful for all her suggestions. And when the College was still nowhere near completing their review by October of 2007, Pat wrote to Dr. Sutcliffe, advising him that she was seriously considering launching a lawsuit against

BCCA. Again, she asked for palpable proof of improvements to their monitoring of Phase 1 human subjects so that she would not have to take such action.

Two months later, she got a reply. It included a copy of the revised consent form, which had gone into effect in February that year. But Dr. Sutcliffe's weak attempt at conciliation came too late. Getting a copy of the official revision, which she had been instrumental in rewording, so many months after it had already been in use, left Pat feeling snubbed.

Meanwhile, none of the lawyers she had spoken with were willing to accept her case as Pat wasn't a "marketable victim." Pat's family lawyer had promised he would help but when he finally approached his firm's litigator, he was too busy. They suggested she go the "self-representation route" in small claims court. This was Pat's only option at that point.

Pat called Eliska, who admitted that running your own lawsuit is daunting. But not impossible. She advised Pat to make sure she had a lawyer who would be willing to read all the required documentation. Using correct legal terminology was critical, she said, and only a lawyer could provide that expertise. In Pat's particular case, there would be an enormous amount of paperwork because there were so many organizations involved. Each doctor would have to be sued individually, as would every institution that was connected in any way, including the provincial government.

Pat made appointments with a couple of local lawyers. Her first meeting was with Ted Holekamp. Sitting across from Mr. Holekamp, she put a simple request to him: to review any of her future legal submissions to make sure she was using the right words. After listening to Pat relate Dave's disastrous clinical trial encounter, Mr. Holekamp responded, "Sure, I'll do it and I'll do it for free!" Receiving this gesture of help, made so quickly and generously after so many months of being dismissed, was too much for Pat to bear. She made her excuses and fled the office in tears.

After calming down, Pat phoned Mr. Holekamp, apologized for her reaction and accepted his kind offer. "Heck," he replied, "I could even drop the writ for you, that'd only cost $289."

Still, Pat hoped that the review of Dave's case by the College might convince BCCA to provide her with solid proof of their revamping of the way Phase 1 recruits were cared for. But December of '07 came and then the New Year was rung in. In the spring of 2008, the long wait — 16 months — for the review of Dave's case by the College ended with the arrival of a letter. The College apologized for the excessive delay and for the fact that they were still unable to locate Dr. Zachary. However, they had decided to issue their report without his input.

"You are most distressed," they wrote, "that in his final hours, your husband was not in a facility that could adequately treat his symptoms in the respectful, compassionate way you wished."

When she read that, Pat was disheartened by the College's lack of perception. She wrote them back: "Possibly, you meant to be solicitous when you state that I was most distressed that my husband spent his final hours in an inadequate, disrespectful facility. But you are way off the mark. My distress stemmed from realizing that Dave was actually dying of the side effects of CPX-1. At no time in the previous week did the BCCA Phase 1 team even hint at that possibility. VGH Emergency was the only adequate, compassionate, respectful medical facility that Dave had the benefit of during his entire association with the trial. I sincerely wish he could have received that high caliber of patient care much earlier in that awful week."

Pat added, "Your report concludes that the College is critical of the care provided to my husband by Dr. Zachary. As well, the College is critical of the communication between Dr. Xavier and Dr. Yvonne. The College has not seen fit to censure these doctors for their failure to communicate with Mr. David Maddocks. I am supposed to be mollified by reports concluding that the days of dithering that preceded and precipitated Dave's death were the result of poor communication between doctors. The only way to combat poor communication is to improve the data collection process. *Careful* observation coupled with concise notations promotes cogent communication; appropriate and timely action can *then* occur. Unfortunately, for Dave and his family, not a single member of the medical Phase I team was '*full of care*.'"

Pat rejected the report as incomplete and asked for copies of the rebuttal letters from the various doctors to substantiate the references made to them in the College's report. She concluded, "I sincerely hope that the College is making a concerted effort to locate Dr. Zachary. Should the College secure a response from Dr. Zachary, I would appreciate being informed. If the College is unable to accomplish this, maybe I could assist by commencing an Internet campaign with the slogan, 'Where in the world is Dr. Zachary?'"

The next month the College located Dr. Zachary; he was working in another province. They said that due to the contents of his rebuttal letter — a letter that the College had pressured Dr. Zachary to provide — and due to Pat's dissatisfaction with their earlier incomplete review, another adjudication would take place.

On September 16, 2008, the Quality of Medical Performance Committee met. This peer review panel of seven physicians and two non-physicians was not a disciplinary committee; it focused instead on remediation of identified concerns.

In the meantime, the College sent Pat copies of the rebuttal letters they'd received from Drs. Xavier, Yvonne and Zachary. Dr. Xavier vehemently maintained that he had been attentive to Dave and had performed his doctoring duties diligently. He stated, "At no point did Mr. or Mrs. Maddocks express concerns about their ability to manage Mr. Maddocks' condition at the Cancer Lodge."[22]

Dr. Yvonne stated that sometime between noon and 1500 hours on December 3, she received a call from the on-call resident regarding Mr. Maddocks, the first time she became aware of him. She went on to say, "He [the resident] sought my opinion as to whether he should be managed as an inpatient or outpatient. I asked about Mr. Maddocks' current hemodynamic status, and any changes in his clinical course compared to previous days. The resident advised me that the only change to his clinical picture was a rise in the creatinine to about 210 from the previous day of about 125. He mentioned that he was clinically stable, not vomiting, keeping fluids down, had normal blood pressure and pulse rate, walked in and out of BCCA under his own strength, and that the frequency of his diarrhea had not changed."[23] Dr. Yvonne said the resident assured her that it was unnecessary for her to come and assess the patient herself.

But the shocker was Dr. Zachary's rebuttal letter to the College. He, too, claimed that his actions had been efficient and solicitous towards Dave on both the Saturday and the Sunday. Dr. Zachary held that it was Dave's large loss of fluid over the previous week, exacerbated by stopping the Imodium, that triggered Dave's irreversible complications. Dr. Zachary pointed out that he had no role in the treatment

22. "The responsibility for the protection of research subjects must always rest with the physician or other health care professional and never [with] the research subject." This is #16 of the Ethical Principles for Medical Research Involving Human Subjects, in the *World Medical Association Declaration of Helsinki*.

23. Pat remembers Dr. Zachary as saying that the creatinine level was 250 but Dr. Yvonne says she was told 210. It was 288. It seems Dr. Yvonne did not question Dr. Zachary about the actual frequency of diarrhea. Upon Dave restarting the Imodium the previous evening, Dr. Zachary's summary stated, "He [Dave] then proceeded to have 1–2 diarrheal movements each hour as was his previous pattern." If extrapolated, the diarrheal movements would then number a possible 24 to 48 times per day surely cause for concern and immediate remedial action. For five days, Dave had not "walked in and out of BCCA under his own strength" but Dr. Zachary stated that he had.

that led to those complications. He then baldly stated, "I was handed a train wreck of a patient by Dr. Xavier who had little to no chance of surviving the weekend." Dr. Zachary went on to list the consequences to himself following the debacle of Dave's death. He claimed that Dr. Xavier, Dr. Yvonne, Dr. O'Reilly, the principal investigator of the trial and his program director berated him to the point that he felt like a "second class citizen." He claimed that "erroneously poor evaluations of subsequent rotations" were deliberate attempts by BCCA to discredit his reputation and led to his losing an oncology job he had been sure he would get with another branch of BCCA. Dr. Zachary claimed "documents prepared by Dr. O'Reilly were cleverly written to minimize culpability regarding Dr. Xavier and Dr. Yvonne but not myself." He further opined that "the physicians at the BCCA and program in general are more concerned about drug company funding and their reputation with industry than the well-being of one of its trainees, or with truth in general." Dr. Zachary also claimed that BCCA's actions towards him had caused him angst in his dealings with the Canadian Medical Protective Association.[24]

On November 12, 2008, the Quality of Medical Performance Committee of the College of Physicians and Surgeons of British Columbia issued Pat its report. The committee was blunt in its indictment of Dr. Xavier's lack of insight — contradicting Dr. Xavier's observation that David Maddocks had "no signs of severe fluid loss." The committee pointed out that "[t]he clearance of edema is an important indication of dehydration." Dr. Xavier was completely aware of this aspect of Dave's decline as he had documented that fact

24. The CMPA is not an insurance company but, rather, offers doctors "assurance" that malpractice defence will be provided during the professional years in which fees are paid. This coverage continues for any issues that may arise after the doctor retires or dies, even though fees are no longer being paid to the CMPA. Doctors pay the CMPA little to no membership fee, as most provincial governments pick up all or some of the tab. The irony is that if you sue a doctor, your tax dollars are likely helping fund his or her lawyers.

a full five days before Dave's death. However, it seems he did not appreciate its significance.

The committee concurred with the conclusions of Dr. Connors, Chairman of the BCCA Research Ethics Board, "that the Phase I program study physicians were unaware of Mr. Maddocks' clinical situation and should have been involved."

They went on. "The committee, therefore, was critical of the care provided by Drs. Xavier, Yvonne and Zachary." As well, "The committee opined that your husband's care deficiencies were not the result of one physician's lack of care, but rather the result of a chain of physician performance and systemic failures, each of which contributed."

None of that was enough for Pat. In a letter back to the Quality of Medical Performance Committee, she wrote: "You will understand that I have little faith that Phase I researchers will remain mindful of their obligation to care for the altruistic volunteers who are the cornerstone upon which modern medicine is built."

"The care protocols applicable to my husband's medical situation were in place — clear and specific. Those protocols were ignored, and as a result, Dave and I were abandoned. You addressed the physicians' failure to perform. But the College's process can never be of assistance to a patient who has suffered the indignities of neglect."

Her fight to get justice for Dave from the Phase I team seemed over. But Pat wasn't finished; she could still help fulfill Dave's wish to be of benefit to others with cancer by doing something to improve the Phase I process for volunteers.

On the advice of her nephew, Jason, a cardiac nurse, Pat started a national registered charitable organization, the Bear Ring "U" 'n Mind Foundation, to advocate for Phase I volunteers and to educate the public about the existence of these heroic people. The Foundation was set up for terminally ill people, neither to recruit them to nor dissuade them from enrolling in such trials, but to supply them with "compassionate, useful information, practical physical assistance and self-help tools."

A major part of that service is a free, private nursing support program called *Research *with* Respect*, provided by Bayshore Home Health Inc., to improve the quality of life for these volunteers during their "away from home" component of a Phase I cancer clinical trial.

"We believe that people dying of cancer who participate in a Phase I clinical trial must be proactive in safeguarding their own physical welfare," says Pat. *Research *with* Respect* (R*w*R) appreciates that Phase I subjects are extremely ill and often far away from home and their normal support base. The Foundation and *R*w*R* exist to inform and assist those amazingly altruistic Phase I volunteers."

Pat's work with R*w*R is ongoing. For more information on her efforts to improve life for Phase I volunteers and their families, please see Appendix C on page 195, or visit the *R*w*R* website: **www.researchwithrespect.ca**.

AFTERWORD

It's Just Business

Thank you for reading *Lethal Dose*.

There are a myriad of messages that Dave's "miserable experience" can bring home to us, for Dave's end-of-life story has implications that reverberate far beyond his close circle of family and friends. True, his is a story about how the medical research industry can fail the volunteers it recruits for cancer clinical trials. But it's also a story about citizenship and community, about ordinary people helping other ordinary people. There are many folks out there like Dave, who have made, and are making, huge — and silent — contributions to our lives.

Whether the violation of vulnerable members of our society generates revulsion or reverence, the bottom line is that the advantages of an innovative pharmaceutical industry are undeniable.

My father, for example, is in his 90s and still enjoys living, thanks to heart medications. My grandsons have survived numerous asthma attacks, thanks to inhalers. My sister-in-law is a 10-year survivor of breast cancer, thanks to chemotherapy. My list, and I'm sure your list, of people who are benefiting from pharmaceuticals is quite lengthy. But it isn't often that we think about, or discuss, how all these life-saving drugs come to be available to us.

The fact is that *all* prescription medications become available because of people like Dave. We live longer, healthier lives because many like him were willing to donate their living bodies to science. And yet, our society doesn't acknowledge, or honour, the contributions they make, and worse, people who do benefit don't seem to care what these volunteers suffer through. I sincerely believe society's — *our* — gross lack of consideration and kindness towards Phase I volunteers stems from our complete ignorance of their existence.

We are not alone in this cluelessness. Indeed, I have found that most medical professionals, including oncology nurses, are unaware of the basic demands made on a Phase I volunteer and are totally oblivious of the ultimate aim of a Phase I trial. The next time you are chatting with a doctor or nurse, or talking with family or friends, introduce the topic of Phase I cancer clinical trials. After reading *Lethal Dose*, you will probably be the only "clued-in" person in the conversation.

Of course, some medical professionals are knowledgeable about the investigational drug process. A liver specialist I am acquainted with, who is involved in testing new drugs, asked me about the *Research *with* Respect* (*R*w*R*) program and Dave's involvement with the Phase I trial. This doctor then solemnly assured me that *he* refuses to participate in any Phase I contracts solely because of the certainty that his physician's oath — Do No Harm — will be broken; he only conducts Phase 2 and 3 clinical trials. Of course, I had to point out the hypocrisy of his stance. He, like a lot of us, directly builds his life and livelihood on the generosity of Phase I volunteers. In fact, we all promote and condone the Phase I process.[25]

By 2030, according to the World Health Organization, half of the world's population will receive a diagnosis of cancer. For today's cancer victims and those of the future, their having a chance to fight and possibly beat this hydra-headed disease depends on volunteers like Dave. This applies,

---

25. What this liver specialist considered to be the ultimate unforgiveable affront was that Dave was required to pay his own parking fees during the away-from-home portion of the CPX-1 trial!

across the board, to all physical and mental maladies requiring medical intervention. But *Lethal Dose* is not about the search for remedies to disease, it is about the people who are helping to fight cancer as Phase I volunteers.

PHARMACEUTICAL ROULETTE

A Phase I clinical trial — the modern version of Russian roulette — is the first time an experimental medical product is used on a human being. In bringing a new drug to the marketplace, a Phase I clinical trial is conducted to find the lowest dose that would cause death. Once that is known, the "safe" dose can be determined and the test drug can move on to Phase 2, in which researchers look at whether that "safe" dose is actually effective. In Phase 3, the goal is to determine whether the new drug is better than medications currently in use. It is in a Phase 3 clinical trial where randomized testing occurs and where the use of placebos could be incorporated. However, in cancer clinical trials, international guidelines forbid the use of placebos. Even so, US researchers are poised to ignore that particular stricture.

If the investigational product being tested proves successful in all these three mandatory phases of clinical trials, then it will likely receive permission to be sold to the public. In Canada, the Therapeutic Products Directorate of Health Canada is the licensing authority; in the USA, it is the Food and Drug Administration or FDA.

In a Phase I cancer trial, the volunteer human subject doesn't have to have a specific type of cancer; they just have to be dying of the cancer they do have. Usually, fewer than 30 subjects are recruited into a Phase I clinical trial. There are groups, known as cohorts, of three or four subjects within each Phase I trial. The individual members of a cohort are not necessarily dealt with by one institution, as a trial can be conducted at other sponsor-contracted sites — certainly in different provinces and often in different countries. In any case, the members of a cohort are not likely to ever meet one another.

The first cohort is given an amount of the experimental drug that lab animals were able to survive.[26] If volunteers in the first cohort have manageable or no side effects, then another cohort is recruited and they are given a higher dose. Throughout the trial, each cohort continues with the dosage that they originally received. More cohorts are recruited; dosages are increased, as per the escalating dose schedule set by the sponsor of the trial and approved by the Research Ethics Board (REB) of the contracted institution. This regimen continues until a human subject experiences severe side effects or death due to the test drug. Then Phase 1 of the trial is stopped.The "safe" dose is deemed to be one or two doses lower than the one that stopped the trial. With enough funding and interest, Phase 2 would then begin. Eighty percent of all clinical trials are sponsored by pharmaceutical companies; the other 20 percent are sponsored by public entities. It should be noted that in a Phase 2 and 3 cancer clinical trial, the human subjects must have the type of cancer that the test drug was designed to combat.

Dave was in the sixth cohort of the Phase 1 trial of CPX-1. After his death, the fourth cohort was deemed to have received the "safe" dose, but upon additional testing of the amount given the fifth cohort, that dosage was then designated as the maximum tolerated "safe" dose or MTD.

If people understood what Dave and people like him endure, if they understood the mental and physical hardships inherent in Dave's faithfully complying with the debilitating demands of a Phase 1 trial, if they knew how stressful it was for him to move to a distant city — with no outside assistance of any kind — for 30 days in the last days of his life, then maybe Phase 1 volunteers would get some respect.

---

26. In August of 2009, Pat was introduced to the manager of the department responsible for the welfare of laboratory animals used in the research centre of a large university. He assured her that these creatures are given the utmost care, in large part because they are valuable. As an example, he told her that each genetically modified mouse is worth $462.

Until society acknowledges its obligations to human subjects in clinical trials, it seems that a small group of friends and I are the only ones willing to act as their advocates and provide practical help. Through our national charitable foundation, we are informing the general public and the medical community that these volunteers need to receive much better care than what is currently in place.

Dave and I, lulled by the rhetoric of the Subject Information and Consent Form, assumed effective monitoring procedures were in place. It turns out that it was my job to advocate for his nutrition and well-being. And, I admit it, I was woefully unprepared and untrained in the role of an overseer and guardian of a human test subject in a Phase I medical experiment. There needs to be a competent third party whose only agenda is to defend the welfare and dignity of Phase I test subjects. Dave never had that.

What Needs to Change

CARING FOR TRIAL VOLUNTEERS

As Dave's story illustrates, participating in a Phase I cancer clinical trial can be a very dehumanizing process. But was his a "one-off" experience? That question is difficult to answer because of the veil of secrecy and confidentiality that surrounds Phase I studies. Occasionally, a case makes the news.[27] The movie *Wit*, starring Emma Thompson as a clinical trial subject with ovarian cancer, dramatizes the indifference to the well-being of trial participants thaat we have found is not unusual. That needs to change. Not only do we need to make the

27. In March 2009, Pat contacted Pamela Fayerman, medical reporter for *The Vancouver Sun*, in an effort to promote *RwR*. Subsequently, on August 19, 2009, *The Sun* published a lengthy article featuring Ms. Anita Cochrane, a young accountant dying of ovarian cancer, who had participated in an early cohort recruited for the Phase 1 trial of ARRY-380. Sometime later, Ms. Fayerman's blog, "Medicine Matters," sadly noted the death of the brave Ms. Cochrane. The March 8/11 edition of MAIL Online, part of the *Daily Mail*, reported Andy Witney's clinical trial experience, which was eerily similar to Dave's ordeal.

organizations involved in these trials live up to their promises to care for these volunteers and provide them with optimal care and attention, we need to have some way to guarantee that.

Some of you may have had experience with a terminally ill person who decided to die at home rather than in hospital. You will be aware of the many services supplied to smooth this very stressful path. Dave and I were astounded by the compassion displayed by our home community. But all that support and caring disappeared when we moved from our home on Vancouver Island to the city of Vancouver for the Phase I trial.

Our Bear Ring "U" 'n Mind Foundation's outreach program provides free, personalized care to a volunteer human subject during their away-from-home period in a Phase I cancer clinical trial. In conjunction with Bayshore Home Health Inc., this nation's largest provider of medical home care services, with more than 8,000 employees, we have developed the clinical support program *Research *with* Respect* (*R*w*R*).

Through this national program, a registered nurse will make a daily visit to the Phase I cancer clinical trial volunteer. That nurse's sole focus is to assure the trial participant's well-being. Additionally, the trial volunteer will have access to 24-hour telephone support from a Bayshore nurse and can receive 60 hours of respite care from a care aide. The *R*w*R* program offers total patient confidentiality. Our foundation receives no information about the patient, just the bill. For information or to access *R*w*R*, phone this toll free number: 866 265-1920.

The Bear Ring "U" 'n Mind Foundation, with its free *Research *with* Respect* program for Phase I cancer volunteers, is a privately funded advocacy group. It was created for the sole purpose of assisting Phase I clinical cancer trial volunteers and has no affiliation with pharmaceutical companies or the research industry. For more information, please check us out online at www.researchwithrespect.ca.

MAKING CLINICAL TRIALS PUBLIC

A Public Clinical Trials Registry is a central repository / list of key information about clinical trials. It must be a "not-for-profit" registry, with free and open access to researchers, clinicians and the general public.

Quote from the Sri Lankan Registry

The Subject Information and Consent Form that Dave and I signed stated, "Since there is very little information about the drug's effect on cancer in humans, we do not expect that you will benefit from taking part in this study, although *the knowledge gained may benefit others.*" (italics added)

As with several other promises of action made to us in that document, the actual delivery mechanisms proved to be less than efficient. But to be fuzzy about *how* the "knowledge gained" is to be shared is shameful.

To "benefit others" is society's *only* vaguely justifiable reason for asking a terminally ill cancer patient to become a human test subject for a Phase I trial of a drug, especially when that drug is not designed for their particular cancer. Any other reason is spurious. But, as the Canadian medical research industry is under no governmental obligation to publish the results of a clinical trial or even to let the general research community know that a trial ever took place, there is no way to know whether the volunteer's efforts *could be* of benefit to others. For society to break faith with a Phase I volunteer in this way is a disgrace.

A bench researcher working on diabetes at the University of Alberta told me that it is absolutely no problem for her to get information on investigational drugs that work; pharmaceutical companies and their stockholders are eager to publish good news. However, in her research, what she needs to know is what *doesn't* work, and that information is not as readily available.

But what is even more appalling than the possibility of non-publication of trial results is that the research community might not even know that a clinical trial took place.

A giant step towards promoting accountability and transparency in the conduct of clinical trials has been made by the International Committee of Medical Journal Editors, ICMJE. Influential publications such as *The Lancet* and *The New England Journal of Medicine,* which these editors represent, are important to the marketing success of any new drug. Drug company reps get instant credibility for their wares when physicians are presented with drug data published in such prestigious magazines. In 2005, the ICMJE decreed that it would not publish drug data if the trial had not first been registered on a public clinical trials registry — *before* the trial began.

In 2006, the World Health Organization got on board with its International Clinical Trials Platform, setting the standard for information that must be submitted on every national public registry being established.

In 2007, the medical editors of the ICMJE toughened their policy, insisting that *all* clinical trials — including Phase I — must be publicly registered before they would publish a drug's data. Pharmaceutical companies can be loath to register their Phase I clinical trials, fearing that proprietary rights might be infringed upon, but the stricter ICMJE position is gradually changing that attitude. But then, not all medical journals are as conscientious as those of the ICMJE, so there are options for sidestepping what some pharmaceutical companies might view as a marketing roadblock.

CREATING A CANADIAN REGISTRY

Health Canada encourages sponsors of clinical trials to register on a public registry of their choice. This is usually the American one, clinicaltrials.gov, but they could register on one in the UK, China, Netherlands, India or Iran, among others. The point is that Health Canada does not actually *require* a pharmaceutical company's clinical trial to be publicly registered, let alone on a *specific* public registry. And so there is no one place where you, your doctor or a researcher can go to access a complete list of every phase of every clinical trial for every disease or condition taking place here in Canada. And, as there is no French language public registry anywhere, that portion of the Canadian citizenry is not served at all.

In Sydney, Australia, I've had a couple of meetings with Dr. Lisa Askie, manager of the Australia New Zealand Clinical Trials Registry, ANZCTR. That national registry was established in 2005. Dr. Askie said that it cost those two countries $250,000 to set up the registry and $500,000 annually to maintain it — remarkably reasonable in the scheme of national programs. She tells me that the number of clinical trials conducted in those two countries is on par with the medical research industry's activity in Canada. Canada is the world's fifth largest biomedical researcher. Dr. Askie assures me that the ANZCTR would be more than willing to assist Canada in establishing its own registry and would be willing to share, at no expense, its computer programs. And if need be, they would consider providing an exclusive Canadian portal on the ANZCTR.

For three years, the Bear Ring "U" 'n Mind Foundation has attempted to ascertain why Canada does not have a Public Clinical Trials Registry. For two of those years, Health Canada said they were studying the idea, "looking for a Canadian approach."[28] Late in 2009, I was told that Canada *will not establish* a registry because creating a new one is frowned upon by the World Health Organization (WHO).

Dr. Askie urged me to connect with Dr. Davina Ghersi at the WHO. Dr. Ghersi had been instrumental in establishing the ANZCTR and had moved over to the WHO to work on their International Clinical Trials Registry Platform or ICTRP.

---

28. The Health Canada website says the idea is still under review. However, late in 2009, an email reply to our foundation from a senior policy analyst with the Therapeutics Products Directorate of HC stated Canada would not establish a public registry. This position taken by HC was confirmed in conversation with two frustrated HC executives at an information session held at the downtown Vancouver campus of SFU in November of 2010.

The WHO website states: "The ICTRP is a country-led initiative. Clinical trial registration happens when countries seek to improve the transparency of clinical trial research involving nationals of that country, and to be more accountable to the individuals who consent to participate in clinical research, and to better oversee and monitor that research. It is up to each country to decide if they want a clinical trial registry."

In her email reply, Dr. Ghersi assured me that a Canadian registry, especially as it would naturally have a French language component, would certainly be welcome. I passed this information on to Health Canada. They asked me to keep them informed about anything else I was able to learn, but HC remains adamant that Canada will not establish a clinical trials registry.

We Need Your Help

CHANGING HEALTH CANADA'S STANCE

A comprehensive listing of all clinical trials occurring in Canada will go a long way towards the following:

- Preventing duplication of research projects, thereby saving time, money and physical and intellectual resources, and reducing the possibility that a human subject's life will be needlessly compromised.
- Providing Canadians with the opportunity to "shop" effectively for cutting-edge medical treatments.
- Achieving the transparency and accountability of an industry that we, having unstintingly funded it through our tax and donation dollars, are entitled to full knowledge of.

According to the National Cancer Institute, less than 20 percent of cancer drugs that go through the Phase 1 trial process ever get to market. A full 70 percent that enter Phase 2 fail to enter Phase 3. Of those that enter Phase 3, 59 percent fail. Moving from Phase 1 to 3 often takes more than a decade.

Without access to information about all these failed trials, the whole trial system becomes risky, inefficient and almost useless.

As Dr. Anthony Robbins, co-editor of the *Journal of Public Health Policy*, has said, "We must not rely on individual morals or societal ethics to protect the public. Rules, regulations and enforcement must be one step ahead of those willing to harm people for financial gain."

With knowledge comes awareness, which in turn promotes appreciation and gratitude. Also, with newly awakened awareness comes personal responsibility with the probability that action will be taken. No doubt this last aspect of knowledge is why the cry "I didn't want to know!" is a common reaction to new information. Truly, I thoroughly understand that feeling. However, your newly acquired appreciation of Phase I cancer clinical trial volunteers and all human subjects participating in medical experiments can be easily and painlessly demonstrated.

WHAT CAN YOU DO?

1. Write a letter to the federal and provincial health ministers advocating for a Canadian Public Clinical Trials Registry or print off the petition letter from our website. No stamp is necessary on letters to the federal government. A copy of the petition letter on the *Research *with* Respect* website can be found in Appendix A of this book. A list of addresses for the relevant government ministries is provided on our website. Send a copy of your letter to your local MP and MLA to keep them in the loop.

2. Read this book and pass it on to others. Please spread the word about the spirit of service that guides Phase I volunteers like Dave.

3. When you make a donation of your money or your time to any organization that funds medical research, ask if that organization actively supports the call for the establishment of a Canadian Public Clinical Trials Registry. If they are not

supportive, find out why. At the very least, make sure that all phases of medical experiments on human beings that you are helping to facilitate are being registered on some public registry somewhere in the world.

4. If there is a hospital in your community, find out whether the hospital's ethics committee has a defined policy regarding public registration of clinical trials. Phase 2 and Phase 3 clinical trials are commonly contracted out to hospitals in smaller centres. Ask if their ethics committee requires the sponsor of any trial operating out of that institution to provide proof that a trial has been publicly registered. If you are told no clinical trials are conducted, then suggest that the board crystallize a policy forthwith so that, should an opportunity to obtain such a contract arise, the hospital's position is clear. Ask, too, whether that institution supports the call for a Canadian Public Clinical Trials Registry. If so, ascertain the actions they have taken; if not, ask why not.

5. Currently there are 10 cities in Canada where Phase 1 cancer clinical trials are conducted: Vancouver, Kelowna, Calgary, Edmonton, London, Mississauga, Ottawa, Toronto, Montreal and Halifax. Find out which hospitals and universities are involved — searching www.clinicaltrials.gov is one way. Ask the research ethics boards (REBs) of these institutions whether they require all trials to be publicly registered and on which registry. Ask if their REB requires the sponsors of clinical trials to publish the results, and ascertain the time frame for publication. Also ask the REB to articulate their position on the establishment of a Canadian Public Clinical Trials Registry.

6. Rescue response teams — such as paramedics, police, firefighters and hospital emergency staff in the above-mentioned cities where Phase 1 away-from-home human subjects are residing as outpatients — should demand that cancer research facilities provide Phase 1 subjects with identification

of their Phase I involvement and the contact number of the trial's principal investigator. The trial subject's DNR status is not relevant at the point of crisis. In order to achieve the scientific goal of a Phase I trial, healthcare providers must be able to officially ascertain whether the subject's serious adverse event is due to the test drug or the subject's underlying disease.

7. We consider the establishment of a Canadian Public Clinical Trials Registry to be a logical first step towards guaranteeing that trial data will be published. Once organized nationally, international initiatives could be achieved with relative ease. There is also the Ottawa Group, an international organization of institutions and individuals focusing on promoting registration of all clinical trials with a strong emphasis on mandatory publication of trial results. The Ottawa Group's ethical rationale states that, "Above all, international trial registration is necessary to fulfill ethical obligations to research participants. When members of the public agree to participate in trials, it is on the understanding that they are contributing to the global body of health-related knowledge. It is thus unethical to conduct human research without ensuring that valid descriptions of the study and its findings are publicly available." Consider adding your or your organization's support to the Ottawa Group: http://ottawagroup.ohri.ca.

The above initiatives are concrete ways for you to express your concern for Phase I cancer clinical trial volunteers and your appreciation of their heroic actions. Your defence of them may, ultimately, be of great benefit to you and yours.

APPENDIX A
Your Chance to Take Action

MAKE YOUR VOICE HEARD ON THESE IMPORTANT POLICY ISSUES:

- Mandatory registration of ALL clinical trials conducted in Canada.
- Registration of clinical trials on any specific country's public registry, as a stop-gap measure until the below occurs.
- Establishment of Canada's own bilingual public registry of clinical trials.

CONTACT THE FEDERAL MINISTER OF HEALTH BY SENDING THE LETTER ON PAGES 188–89 TO:

The Minister of Health
Health Canada
Brooke Claxton Building
Tunney's Pasture
Ottawa, Ontario K1A 0K9
Locator #0906C
(No postage required on the envelope)

DEAR HONOURABLE MINISTER OF HEALTH

Recently, through *Research *with* Respect*, a program of the Bear Ring "U" 'n Mind Foundation, I have been made aware of how Phase I cancer clinical trials are conducted in Canada. I am writing directly to you to convey my alarm and concern with the lack of effective organization and regulation inherent in our present system of clinical trials.

I am dismayed that Canada **does not** have its own national Clinical Trials Registry, available in both official languages, and that those involved in the medical research industry — researchers, doctors, pharmaceutical companies — are not required to post basic identifying information on their studies on a publicly available site, not even for the riskiest of trials, the Phase I clinical trial. As well, they are **not** required to post information on the public clinical trial registries of other countries. Many Canadians are unaware of this lapse in safety; and if they were aware, they would consider it reprehensible.

As you know, a Phase I cancer clinical trial discerns the safety margins of an investigational treatment. It is a dangerous undertaking and the motivation for many citizens is one of unselfishness and generosity: knowing that their own medical condition is terminal, they agree to offer themselves as test subjects to determine safe dosage, subsequent to the completion of experiments on lab animals.

Phase I volunteers want their legacy to be that they made a difference. They hope that the knowledge gained will help others. They place their trust in researchers, anticipating they will be treated ethically and fairly. We must not let them down.

If you as Minister of Health establish mandatory registration of all clinical trials on a Public Clinical Trials Registry, then all stakeholders — researchers, medical practitioners and the public — would have a beginning point to ascertain clinical trial activity and subsequent findings. Duplication of international research efforts would be eliminated. And human lives might be saved.

I urge you to move to protect these vulnerable members of our society, the terminally ill, by providing the accountability and transparency of a Public Clinical Trials Registry.

I look forward to hearing your comments on this important and urgent issue.

Date: ______________________________

Signature: ______________________________

Printed Name: ______________________________

Address: ______________________________

APPENDIX B
CPX-1 Report Card

The information for this appendix came from various inteviews and websites.

CPX-1 is the combination of two cancer drugs, Irinotecan HCI and Floxuridine, often used in the treatment of colorectal cancer. Both drugs have had success treating cancer, particularly gastrointestinal tumours and advanced colorectal cancer. CPX-1 combines the two in a fat liposome; Celator's use of the fat liposome represents a new drug delivery strategy for cancer treatment. However, this innovative method intensifies the drugs' effects, so rigorous testing is required.

Traditionally, drugs such as Irinotecan HCI and Floxuridine have been administered as a saline-based cocktail that floods the whole body. Since the strength of each component in the cocktail wanes at different rates, it requires a fine balancing act to determine a dosage that provides the maximum synergistic benefit. The intended outcome of delivering the drugs within a fat liposome is to achieve a heightened, constant and consistent effect of the combined drugs on the body.

Mark Dewhirst, professor of radiation oncology at Duke University Medical Center, says, "Encapsulating the drugs inside of fat liposomes and infusing them into the bloodstream enables us to deliver 30 times more chemotherapy than we normally could to the tumour site ... The liposomes melt only within the tumour, and the rest of the body receives relatively less of the toxic drug."[29] Dr. Dewhirst refers to adjusting drugs that are already widely used. Reusing extensively prescribed cancer drugs and combining one or more of them in a cutting-edge approach is the basis for a large portion of cancer research currently underway. The possibility of duplication

29. http://her2support.org/vbulletin/archive/index.php/t-26560.html

is high, which is precisely why mandatory public registration (preferably on a Canadian registry) and mandatory publication of all clinical trials is vital.

There were 33 human participants in the multi-site Phase I trial of CPX-1; 15 of the 33 had advanced colorectal cancer. The published trial data summary stated that 72.7 percent of those 15 showed "clinical benefit, including partial tumour regression or stable disease." A 5.4-month delay of disease progression was noted. These encouraging numbers are applicable only to this colorectal sub-group, which represents less than half of the recruited volunteers.

Based on the Phase I findings, Celator went ahead with Phase 2, using only test subjects diagnosed with advanced colorectal cancer — the type of cancer that CPX-1 was actually designed to combat. In June 2008, they completed the Phase 2 trial with 59 volunteers. The starting dose, established by the Phase I trial, produced "higher than expected adverse events and treatment discontinuations. This resulted in higher than expected dose reductions and treatment delays."[30]

Only 20 percent of Phase I drugs ever get approved and make it to market; 80 percent go nowhere. It appears that CPX-1 has become one of the 80 percent of drugs that don't successfully complete the obligatory three phases of clinical trials. The safe dosage proved to be unsafe; should further studies be attempted, they will be conducted at a lower dosage.

According to its website, Celator is currently seeking a partner to further the clinical development of CPX-1, but there are no open clinical trials with the drug; it never made it past Phase 2. Celator's website states: "This study is ongoing, but not recruiting participants." Celator should, however, be commended for providing the research community with a clear picture of the CPX-1 studies.

Dave's death occurred at the highest prescribed dosage. No one since has received that dose.

30. http://www.celatorpharma.com/new/files/poster_cpx1_WCGIC2008_Batist.pdf

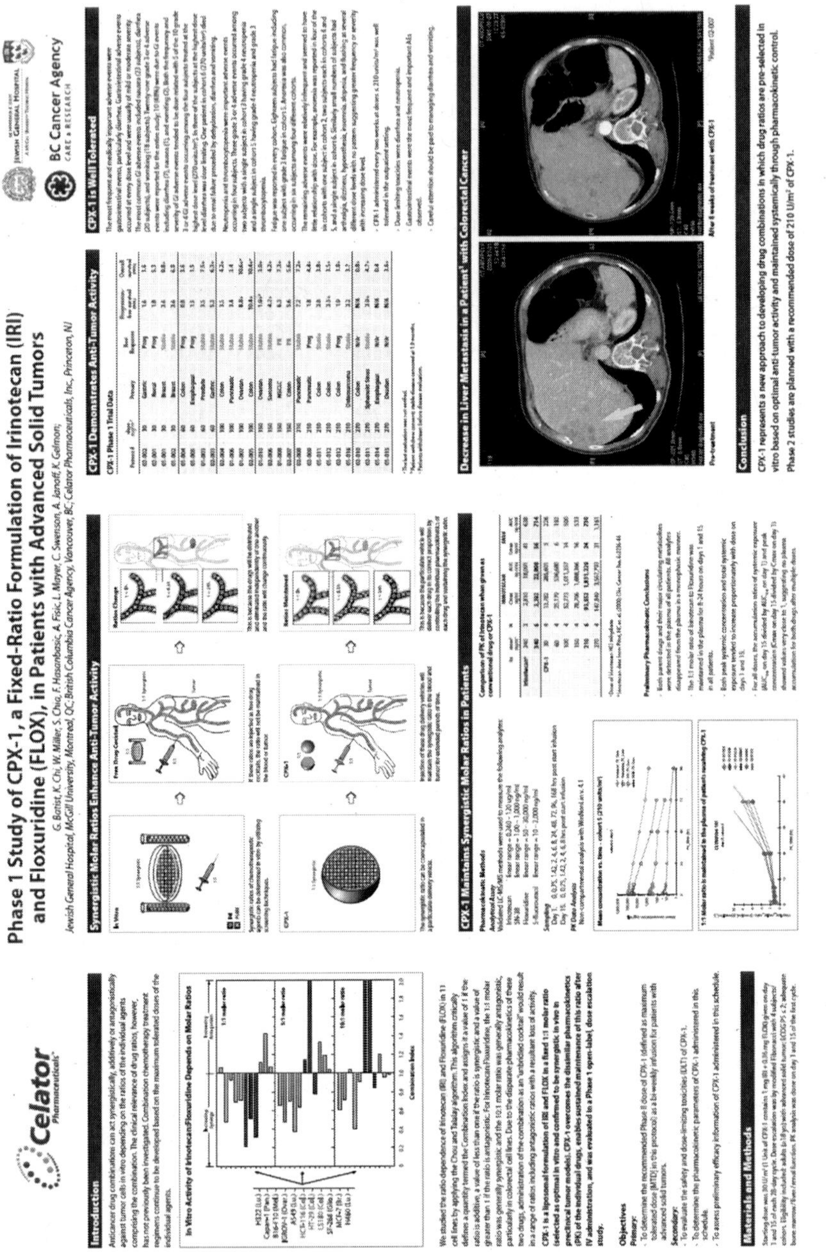

"Celator Pharmaceuticals Publications," last modified August 16, 2011, http://www.celatorpharma.com/new/publications_cpx1.html

From *Phase 1 Study of CPX-1,*
a Fixed-Ratio Formulation of Irinotecan (IRI) and Floxuridine (FLOX), in Patients with Advanced Solid Tumors
(Seen on Opposite Page)

CPX-1 Demonstrates Anti-Tumor Activity

CPX-1 Phase 1 Trial Data

Patient #	dose mg/m^2	Primary	Best Response	Progression-free survival (mos.)	Overall survival (mos.)
02-002	30	Gastric	Prog	1.6	1.6
02-001	30	Renal	Prog	1.8	5.3
01-001	30	Breast	Stable	3.6	9.8+
01-002	30	Breast	Stable	3.6	6.9
01-004	60	Colon	Prog	0.8	3.6
01-005	60	Esophageal	Prog	1.5	1.5
01-003	60	Prostate	Stable	3.5	7.5+
02-003	60	Gastric	Stable	5.3	6.3+
02-004	100	Colon	Stable	3.5	4.2+
01-006	100	Pancreatic	Stable	3.4	3.4
01-007	100	Ovarian	Stable	8.8+	10.6+[a]
02-005	100	Colon	Stable	10.4+	10.4+[a]
01-010	150	Ovarian	Stable	1.9+[b]	3.0+
02-006	150	Sarcoma	Stable	4.2+	4.2+
01-008	150	NSCLC	PR	6.3	7.3+
02-007	150	Colon	PR	5.6	5.6+
02-008	210	Pancreatic	Stable	7.2	7.2+
02-009	210	Pancreatic	Prog	1.8	4.4+
01-011	210	Colon	Stable	3.8	3.8+
01-012	210	Colon	Stable	3.5+	3.5+
02-012	210	Colon	Prog	1.9	1.9+
01-016	210	Osteosarcoma	Stable	3.2	3.7
02-010	270	Colon	N/A[c]	N/A	0.8+
02-011	270	Sphenoid Sinus	Stable	3.9+	4.7+
01-014	270	Esophageal	N/A[c]	N/A	0.4
01-015	270	Ovarian	N/A[c]	N/A	3.6+

[a] The last evaluation was not verified.
[b] Patient withdrew consent; stable disease censored at 1.9 months.
[c] Patients withdrawn before disease evaluation.

CPX-1 is Well Tolerated

The most frequent and medically important adverse events were gastrointestinal events, particularly diarrhea. Gastrointestinal adverse events occurred at every dose level and were usually of mild or moderate severity. The most common GI adverse events included nausea (23 subjects), diarrhea (20 subjects), and vomiting (18 subjects). Twenty-one grade 3 or 4 adverse events were reported for the entire study; 10 (48%) were due to GI events including diarrhea (7), nausea (1), and vomiting (2). Both the frequency and severity of GI adverse events tended to be dose related with 5 of the 10 grade 3 or 4 GI adverse events occurring among the four subjects treated at the highest dose level (270 units/m^2). In three of the subjects at the highest dose level diarrhea was dose limiting. One patient in cohort 6 (270 units/m^2) died due to renal failure preceded by dehydration, diarrhea and vomiting.

Neutropenia and thrombocytopenia were important adverse events occurring in four subjects. Three grade 3 or 4 adverse events occurred among two subjects with a single subject in cohort 3 having grade 4 neutropenia and a single subject in cohort 5 having grade 4 neutropenia and grade 3 thrombocytopenia.

Fatigue was reported in every cohort. Eighteen subjects had fatigue including one subject with grade 3 fatigue in cohort 5. Anorexia was also common, occurring in six subjects among four different cohorts.

The remaining adverse events were relatively infrequent and seemed to have little relationship with dose. For example, anorexia was reported in four of the six cohorts with one subject in cohort 2, two subjects each in cohorts 4 and 5, and a single subject in cohort 6. Similarly small numbers of subjects had arthralgia, dizziness, hypoesthesia, insomnia, alopecia, and flushing at several different dose levels with no pattern suggesting greater frequency or severity with increasing dose level.

- CPX-1 administered every two weeks at doses ≤ 210 units/m^2 was well tolerated in the outpatient setting.
- Dose limiting toxicities were diarrhea and neutropenia.
- Gastrointestinal events were the most frequent and important AEs observed.
- Careful attention should be paid to managing diarrhea and vomiting.

APPENDIX C
About *Research *with* Respect*

*Research *with* Respect* is a free-to-the-client outreach support program for Phase I cancer clinical trial volunteers, provided by the national charitable organization Bear Ring "U" 'n Mind Foundation. This is an independent foundation with no connection to the pharmaceutical or medical research industries. Free, private nursing services are provided by Bayshore Home Health and all funding comes entirely from private citizens, some of whose loved ones have been Phase I clinical cancer trial volunteers.

*Research *with* Respect* seeks to improve the monitoring and care given to Phase I clinical trial subjects, who must agree to relocate near the research facility for the first month of a trial. The trials are conducted on an outpatient basis. The foundation recognizes that such a relocation requirement is a huge demand of these very ill people and their worried families.

*Research *with* Respect* provides the following services during the away-from-home period:

- Daily visit by a Bayshore Home Health nurse
- Pain and symptom management review
- Client education
- Emotional support
- Liaison with cancer research centres

*Research *with* Respect* is currently available in Vancouver and Toronto. A Phase I cancer clinical trial client requesting *RwR* in any other Canadian city should give Bayshore Home Health one week notice.

For more information, or to register for services, call toll free **1 866-265-1920,** or visit *Research *with* Respect* online at www.researchwithrespect.ca/.

"At the point of dying,
the issue will not be that
we die but how we die."

Therese A. Rondo